DEVELOPMENT IN PRACTICE

Enriching Lives

Enriching Lives

Overcoming Vitamin and Mineral Malnutrition in Developing Countries

THE WORLD BANK
WASHINGTON, D.C.

The Development in Practice series publishes reviews of the World
Bank's activities in different regions and sectors. It lays particular
emphasis on the progress that is being made and on the policies and
practices that hold the most promise of success in the effort to reduce
poverty in the developing world.

The findings, interpretations, and conclusions expressed in this
study are entirely those of the authors and should not be attributed in
any manner to the World Bank, to its affiliated organizations, or to
members of its Board of Executive Directors or the countries they
represent.

Library of Congress Cataloging-in-Publication Data

Enriching lives : overcoming vitamin and mineral malnutrition in
    developing countries.
        p.   cm. — (Development in practice)
    Includes bibliographical references.
    ISBN 0-8213-2987-1
    1. Malnutrition—Developing countries.   2. Avitaminosis—
Developing countries.   3. Minerals in human nutrition—Developing
countries.   I. International Bank for Reconstruction and
Development. II. Series: Development in practice (Washington, D.C.)
RA645.N87E57   1994
363.8—dc20   94-27022
                                                            CIP

Contents

Boxes

Figures

Text Tables

Appendix Tables

Foreword

Two years ago, when I was asked to become the Vice President for Human Resources Development and Operations Policy at the World Bank, few people were familiar with the term "micronutrients." Since then, many have learned that vitamin and mineral deficiencies impose high economic costs on virtually every developing country, but that micronutrient programs are among the most cost-effective of all health programs—with high returns in terms of human resources.

World Development Report 1993 highlighted both needs and opportunities. This follow-up book provides the underpinnings—convincing detailed arguments for addressing micronutrient malnutrition and practical advice based on lessons learned from program experience. The messages are clear: educate consumers so that they fully appreciate and understand the importance of micronutrients in the food they eat; encourage fortification of foodstuffs using a combination of market incentives and regulatory enforcement; and, when that still is not enough to meet a population's need, distribute micronutrient capsules and other supplements using all public and private channels available. Public financing may be needed in the short run to launch such an effort and for those groups unable to pay, but over the long run consumers should pay for the necessary vitamins and minerals (less than US$1 per person per year).

Today World Bank–assisted projects in thirty countries have micronutrient components. That is not enough. We propose to encourage cost-effective micronutrient components in every appropriate World Bank project where micronutrient malnutrition exists and is not being addressed by other means. This effort will require greater client ownership and stronger partnerships with nongovernmental organizations, private industry, and bilateral and international agencies. Toward that same goal, we will continue to sponsor—along with the Canadian International Development Agency, the International Development Research Centre, the United Nations International Children's Educational Fund, and the United Nations Development Programme—the Micronutrient Initiative, which the World Bank helped create, as a catalyst of greater action in the affected countries, among donors, and by the food industry.

Armeane M. Choksi
Vice President
Human Resource Development
and Operations Policy
The World Bank

Acknowledgments

THIS paper was prepared by Judith McGuire, PHN (Task Manager), and Rae Galloway (Consultant) from materials prepared by Howard Bouis, John Dunn, Rudolfo Florentino, Wilma Freire, Philip Gowers, Ted Greiner, the International Council for the Control of Iodine Deficiency Disorders, Festo Kavishe, Benny Kodiat, The Manoff Group, Charlotte Neumann, Antonio Pardo, Mario Rivadeneira, Robert Tilden, M. G. Venkatesh Mannar, and Ray Yip. Gregg Forte was the editor.

The team would like to thank the Internal Advisory Committee (Alan Berg, Alain Colliou, Joy De Beyer, Oscar Echeverri, James Greene, Salim Habayeb, and Anthony Measham) and the External Reviewers (David Alnwick, Kenneth Bailey, Martin Bloem, Graeme Clugston, Frances Davidson, Ted Greiner, Peter Greaves, Steven Hansch, Basil Hetzel, E. J. R. Heyward, Abraham Horwitz, Rolf Klemm, Sonya Rabanek, Richard Seifman, Nevin Scrimshaw, Barbara Underwood, M. G. Venkatesh Mannar, Fernando Viteri, and Richard Young) for their insightful comments.

Abbreviations and Acronyms

CGIAR	Consultative Group on International Agricultural Research
DALY	Disability-adjusted life-year
EPI	Expanded Program on Immunization
FAO	Food and Agriculture Organization of the United Nations
GDP	Gross domestic product
ICCIDD	International Council for the Control of Iodine Deficiency Disorders
ICDS	Integrated Child Development Program
IDD	Iodine deficiency disorders
INACG	International Nutritional Anemia Consultative Group
IVACG	International Vitamin A Consultative Group
NGO	Nongovernmental organization
SCN	SubCommittee on Nutrition of the UN Administrative Coordinating Committee
UNICEF	United Nations International Children's Educational Fund
USAID	United States Agency for International Development
WHO	World Health Organization

Executive Summary

THE control of vitamin and mineral deficiencies is one of the most extraordinary development-related scientific advances of recent years. Probably no other technology available today offers as large an opportunity to improve lives and accelerate development at such low cost and in such a short time.

Dietary deficiencies of vitamins and minerals—life-sustaining nutrients needed only in small quantities (hence, "micronutrients")—cause learning disabilities, mental retardation, poor health, low work capacity, blindness, and premature death. The result is a devastating public health problem: about 1 billion people, almost all in developing countries, are suffering the effects of these dietary deficiencies, and another billion are at risk of falling prey to them.

To grasp the enormous implications at the country level, consider a country of 50 million people with the levels of micronutrient deficiencies that exist today in South Asia. Such a country would suffer the following *losses each year* because of these deficiencies:

- 20,000 deaths
- 11,000 children born cretins or blinded as preschoolers
- 1.3 million person-years of work lost due to lethargy or more severe disability
- 360,000 student-years wasted (3 percent of total student body).

In terms of losses by type of deficiency, more than 13 million people suffer night blindness or total blindness for the lack of vitamin A. In areas without adequate iodine in the diet, five to ten offspring of every 1,000 pregnant women are dead upon birth or soon thereafter due to iodine deficiency. Severe iron deficiency causes as many as one in five maternal deaths, as well as the death of about 30 percent of children who enter the hospital with it and do not get a blood transfusion (those who do get the transfusion are exposed to other risks).

1

The World Bank's *World Development Report 1993* found micronutrient programs to be among the most cost-effective of all health interventions. Most micronutrient programs cost less than $50 per disability-adjusted life-year (DALY) gained. Deficiencies of just vitamin A, iodine, and iron—the focus of this book—could waste as much as 5 percent of gross domestic product, but addressing them comprehensively and sustainably would cost less than 0.3 percent of gross domestic product (GDP).

The 1990 Summit for Children endorsed three micronutrient goals for the end of the decade: the virtual elimination of iodine and vitamin A deficiencies and the reduction of iron deficiency anemia in women by one-third. The goals were reaffirmed in 1991 at the Ending Hidden Hunger conference and in 1992 at the International Conference on Nutrition. The goals are achievable only if political will, state-of-the-art technology, and private, public, and international resources are marshaled for the effort.

The Need for a Comprehensive Approach

The alleviation of poverty and the strengthening of national health care systems alone cannot solve the problem of micronutrient deficiencies. Because the micronutrient content of foods is a hidden property, consumers do not automatically demand micronutrient-rich foods with increased income. Thus, food and agriculture policies need to watch over not only the quantity but the nutritional quality of the food supply and promote the production, marketing, and consumption of micronutrient-rich foods. Likewise, safety net programs, including refugee feeding, must respond to the total nutritional needs of target groups and not just to their calorie and protein needs.

An overall improvement in health system management will go a long way toward improving micronutrient malnutrition as long as programs train and monitor medical personnel for the prevention and management of micronutrient deficiencies, reach groups not currently using the health care system, and, through teaching and persuasion, transform consumers into a constituency for healthful diet.

Three Types of Approaches

Even with the most nutritionally enlightened economic development plan, developing countries must still take direct aim at micronutrient malnutrition through consumer education, aggressive distribution of pharmaceutical supplements, and the fortification of common foodstuffs or water.

Fortunately, all of these options are inexpensive and cost-effective. The particular mix of interventions chosen depends on country conditions. But the key constraints to achieving the summit goals are a lack of awareness and commitment of policymakers and consumers, a weak capacity to deliver supplements and education, and a lack of enforcement of industry compliance with fortification laws.

Social Mobilization

Policymakers must be motivated to take action against micronutrient malnutrition. They need persuasive information on the economic and social costs of micronutrient malnutrition and on the political salience and cost-effectiveness of micronutrient programs. Then, during implementation, good management information systems and public education programs designed into the overall initiative can make the public aware of the improvements resulting from the micronutrient programs and draw the connection to the responsible program managers and policymakers. That connection provides public support and reward for the initiative of the political leaders.

Beyond the immediate political feedback they provide, programs to educate, persuade, and change the behavior of consumers are essential to the long-run elimination of micronutrient deficiencies. Subconscious consumer demand for micronutrients needs to be made conscious and directed to appropriate foods and pharmaceuticals. This demand will serve as a "pull" factor to bring the target groups to distribution points for supplements, to overcome resistance, and, if necessary, to induce consumers to pay a little more for a better (that is, a fortified, although unfamiliar) diet. Social marketing of micronutrients and micronutrient-rich foods is necessary in virtually all developing countries, even where health service delivery is good and the food industry is well developed.

Pharmaceutical Supplementation

Two key problems in pharmaceutical supplementation have been poor coverage of at-risk groups and inadequate supply management. To overcome the coverage problem, the delivery of supplements must break out of a single-clinic-based track and employ every possible avenue of convenience and opportunity, including school visits, workplace programs, and nutritional safety net programs.

The goals of supply management are to procure effective supplements that look appealing, have helpful packaging and labeling, come in the right doses, and are affordable; to store and transport them for maximal quality and preservation; and to deliver them to well-selected distribution points in adequate numbers of doses at an appropriate frequency. Achieving these goals requires committed program leaders, motivated and well-trained workers, good monitoring and surveillance, and a demanding public. The private pharmaceuticals market may have an important role to play in developing new products and delivering supplements in a cost-effective manner at the community level.

Effective Regulation and Incentives for the Private Food Industry

The food industry responds to both positive and negative policy signals. Broad legislation, followed by technical regulations, should require micronutrient fortification of basic foodstuffs and support a fair and honest regulatory system that monitors compliance and punishes the noncompliant.

This legislation should be joined by financial and political inducements to industry. Some of the incentives used in effective fortification programs have been tax relief, import licenses, loans for equipment, subsidies on fortificants, and positive press coverage.

A third component of any successful food control system is consumer awareness and pressure for industry compliance. Consumers can be mobilized through social marketing and consumer organizations to demand effective fortification. Without confidence in both the industry and the regulatory apparatus, enlightened consumers will not be willing to buy new products.

Developing Nutritional Awareness and Habits

Political sustainability comes from monitoring and communications as well as satisfaction of consumer demands. One of the greatest advantages of micronutrient programs is that, because results are unambiguously attributable to specific interventions, policymakers can take credit for improvements.

Operational sustainability depends upon good management, continual oversight, the retraining of personnel, and the supervision of delivery systems (particularly the health system and food industry).

Behavioral sustainability will come only after consumers form good nutrition habits, whether that means eating carrots, taking a daily iron pill, or buying a fortified food.

Economic sustainability is a function of national and household ability to pay. Micronutrients are so inexpensive that, regardless of the form, they should ultimately be affordable by the intended beneficiaries. For equity reasons or in the short term, some form of targeted subsidy may be necessary to reach the poorest and to form habits among the desired beneficiaries. In the long run, however, financial sustainability will depend upon consumers' willingness to pay for the nutrients. It is the government's responsibility to choose the most cost-effective means of delivering micronutrients to the population.

The Need for External Start-up Support

Micronutrient interventions are among the most cost-effective investments in the health sector. Because fortification of water and foods is also extremely cost-effective, nontraditional sector involvement is desirable as well. Donors have a key role to play in assisting with program design and financing. Addressing micronutrient deficiencies globally will require an estimated $1 billion per year—about $1 per affected person (all dollar amounts are U.S. dollars). That figure is equivalent to the economic costs of endemic deficiencies of vitamin A, iodine, and iron in *a single country* of 50 million people. Most of these costs will ultimately be borne by consumers when purchasing food with higher nutritional quality.

In the short run, however, donors and governments may have to assume a major financial burden for project preparation, start-up costs, and recurrent costs in the early years. The economic and social payoffs from micronutrient programs reach as high as 84 times the program costs. Few other development programs offer such high social and economic payoffs.

CHAPTER ONE

The Challenge of Dietary Deficiencies of Vitamins and Minerals

THE life and vitality of human beings depend crucially on certain vitamins and minerals that help determine the efficient functioning of the brain, the immune system, reproduction, and energy metabolism. The body needs only small amounts of these nutrients—micrograms or milligrams per day (hence the term micronutrients)—but it cannot manufacture them. They must be part of the diet or taken as supplements. Deficiencies of even the small amounts required cause learning disabilities, impair work capacity, and bring on illness and death. Micronutrient malnutrition is most devastating for pre-school children and pregnant women, but it is debilitating for all ages. And it is debilitating for the national economy as well.

The Strategic Importance of Vitamin A, Iodine, and Iron

Virtually every developing country has a deficiency in vitamin A, iodine, or iron that is large enough to constitute a public health problem; many developing countries have multiple deficiencies.[1] More than 2 billion people worldwide are at risk from deficiencies of these nutrients, and more than 1 billion are actually ill or disabled by them; almost all are in the developing world (Table 1.1).

Unfortunately, the rise in caloric intake that accompanies economic development and higher income does not solve the problem of micronutrient mal-

6

Table 1.1 Population at Risk of and Affected by Micronutrient Malnutrition, by WHO Region, 1991

(millions)[a]

Region	Iodine deficiency disorders		Vitamin A deficiency		Iron-deficient or anemic
	At risk	Affected (goiter)	At risk	Affected (xerophthalmia)[b]	
Africa	150	39	18	1.3	206
Americas	55	30	2	0.1	94
South and Southeast Asia	280	100	138	10.0	616
Europe	82	14	—	—	27
Eastern Mediterranean	33	12	13	1.0	149
Western Pacific and China	405	30	19	1.4	1,058
Total	1,005	225	190	13.8	2,150

— Not available.
a. See Appendix A for further details.
b. Xerophthalmia (drying of the eye) is a general term for all eye signs of severe vitamin A deficiency including blindness. See Appendix A for further details.
Source: WHO 1992.

nutrition—these nutrients are not present in all foods (some are present in very few), and people do not have a natural hunger for them.

On the other hand, there are well-established, low-cost means of prevention and treatment for deficiencies of vitamin A, iodine, and iron in developing countries. The effectiveness of these measures can be clearly measured, and they are the focus of this book.

The dietary sources of the three micronutrients and the consequences of their deficiencies vary:

■   *Vitamin A* is found in fruits and vegetables, liver, and breastmilk. Humans need less than one-thousandth of one gram of it per day, but more than 13 million people suffer night blindness or permanent blindness for lack of it. In areas of endemic deficiency, more than one of every 10,000 children under the age of six is blind. Six of every ten preschool children with severe vitamin A deficiency die.

■   *Iodine* has been depleted from the soil in many parts of the world. In those areas, five to ten offspring of every 1,000 pregnant women who do not eat seafood or otherwise get iodine (such as through iodine-fortified salt) are dead upon birth or soon thereafter (Clugston, Dulberg, Pandav, and Tilden 1987);

many of those who survive are cretins—mentally retarded, spastic, and with low life expectancy. Many others are deaf, mute, or mildly to moderately retarded. Iodine deficiency in adults reduces work potential (Hetzel 1989). More than 200 million people worldwide lack adequate iodine in their diet.

■ *Iron* is found in red meat and breastmilk. It also exists in grains, legumes, and vegetables but in a form less easily absorbed unless taken at the same time with meat or foods rich in vitamin C. Thus diets of grains, legumes, and vegetables in developing countries are often deficient in *absorbable* iron (DeMaeyer 1989). About 1 billion people suffer clinical anemia. Severe anemia causes as many as one in five maternal deaths. Children born of anemic mothers are often stunted and sickly. Severe anemia kills about 30 percent of children who enter the hospital with it and do not get an immediate transfusion of blood; those who do get the transfusion are exposed to other risks (Lakritz, Campbell, and Ruebush II 1992). A less-severe deficiency of iron in the preschool years, even if corrected, permanently reduces the manual dexterity of children, limits their attention span, and shortens their memory capacity (Seshadri and Gopaldas 1989; Lozoff, Jimenez, and Wolf 1991). As with iodine, a deficiency of iron in adults reduces work capacity: in anemic people, a 10 percent increase in hemoglobin (the iron-containing component of blood essential to transport oxygen) of a moderately anemic person raises work output 10 to 20 percent (Levin 1986).

The Scope of Micronutrient Malnutrition

To grasp the costs of nutrient deficiencies, consider a country of 50 million with the level of micronutrient deficiencies that exists today in South Asia. Such a country would suffer the following losses *each year,* due entirely to inadequate vitamin A, iron, and iodine:

■ 20,000 deaths
■ 11,000 children born cretins or blinded as preschoolers
■ 1.3 million person-years of work lost due to lethargy or more severe disability
■ 360,000 student-years wasted.

The monetary cost associated with the personal and social tragedy of these human losses depends on the wage rate and the imputed economic value of a human life. Assuming a conservative estimate of $750 in wages per person-year of work and $1,000 per life lost, the monetary cost of the 1.3 million person-years of work would reach almost $1 billion per year, about $20 per capita. The 20,000 excess deaths per year and the future social burden and wage losses imposed by the lost schooling and physical handicaps of the children add even more to the loss.

To give only one example of the possible return on investment from a program of correction, and to anticipate the discussion in Chapter 2, fortifying the food and water supply with vitamin A, iodine, and iron for all in this country of 50 million would cost about $25 million per year, or $0.50 per capita (versus $20 per capita in the above estimate of annual malnutrition costs); such fortification could virtually eliminate the lost work capacity, blindness, cretinism, and death caused by deficiencies of the targeted micronutrients. The $25 million investment would thus yield a fortyfold *annual* return on investment even without counting the future costs. Even with only a 50 percent coverage of the neediest people in the country, the returns from micronutrient programs vastly outweigh the costs. Put another way, assuming a per capita GDP of $350 ($17.5 billion for the whole country), the current-year losses from micronutrient malnutrition ($1 billion) amount to more than 5 percent of GDP, whereas the $25 million program of fortification costs less than 0.15 percent of GDP (see Appendix B for further discussion).

Beyond the Reach of Economic Development

Poor people are more likely than others to suffer from micronutrient malnutrition; but micronutrient intake does not necessarily improve in step with income, because the micronutrient content of foods is a hidden quality to the uninformed consumer. People know when they are hungry and when they have had enough to eat. They have no natural hunger, however, for vitamin A, iodine, iron, or other micronutrients; they generally do not know that they need them; and they do not know what foods provide them.

The signs that someone hasn't eaten enough of a particular vitamin or mineral are subtle and delayed, and they may not seem severe or diet-related to the victim. Even cretinism and blindness are more likely to be attributed to divine retribution than they are to diet.

Some micronutrients are heavily concentrated in a few foods, so just by eating more or having a more varied diet will not necessarily increase the intake of those micronutrients unless consumer demand has been directed to the right foods. For example, in the absence of fortification, iodine intake can be constant regardless of income because its concentration in food is a function of its concentration in the soil. Only wealthy consumers in iodine-deficient regions may get adequate amounts of iodine because they can afford to buy seafood, food from abroad, and iodized salt.

The intake of vitamin C (which helps in iron absorption) and vitamin A changes only erratically with income. Because these vitamins are concentrated in perishable fruits and dark green, leafy vegetables, their consumption largely depends on agricultural seasons. In rural areas, wild foods contribute a considerable amount of vitamin A to the diet. As income rises, however, the consumption of vitamin A often decreases because traditional foods, including breastmilk, are disdained. With their access to cultivated fruits and dairy products and the refrigeration to keep them, the highest income groups are able to raise the level of vitamins C and A in their diet.

In principle, both the quantity and quality of iron in the diet is related to income.[2] Yet in Asia and Latin America, iron availability in the past twenty to thirty years has declined, perhaps because of a decline of legumes in the diet, while income and caloric intake have generally risen (Figure 1.1). In Africa, income and the supply of food have stagnated, and the supplies of both vitamin A and iron have declined, perhaps because of less reliable supplies of red palm oil (rich in vitamin A) and a dietary shift from grains to tubers. The consumption of vitamin A has risen in Asia largely because of greater supplies of red palm oil, and in Latin America and the Near East because the more diverse diet that has been acquired with higher income has included more vegetables and dairy foods.

Good Health Care Systems: Necessary but Not Sufficient

Vitamin and mineral deficiencies loom as a public health problem in all developing countries. They require preventive measures that go well beyond the function of health care delivery. Of course, good health care systems, important in their own right, can contribute a great deal to the nutritional condition of the population. Hookworm disease, for example, a cause of anemia, should be treated with antihookworm medicine and iron supplements. Vitamin and mineral supplementation is an important part of the care of pregnant women and young children, and it is also vital in the treatment of numerous diseases, including measles, chronic diarrhea, lower respiratory infection, and malaria. Because breastmilk is rich in high-quality vitamin A and iron, breastfeeding promotion should be central to any health care system as well.

The Need for Special Programs

The last few decades in the developing world have shown that serious vitamin and mineral deficiencies are not uniformly corrected by rising income, at least over any acceptable time frame. Although health care programs provide a necessary point of intervention, they cannot completely correct the causes of deficiencies.

Figure 1.1   Changes in Availability of Vitamin A, Iron, and Food Energy by FAO Region from 1960/65 to 1986/88

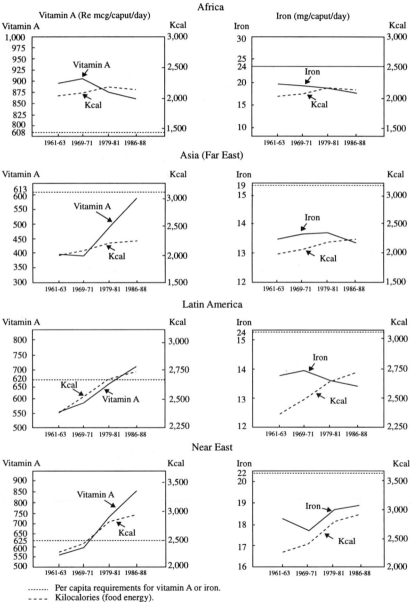

.... Per capita requirements for vitamin A or iron.
- - - - Kilocalories (food energy).
Source: FAO 1992 database (AGROSTAT/PC, Food Balance Sheets, FAO, Rome).

**BOX 1.1 WHEN TO CONSIDER USING
AN IRON PROGRAM**

Iron deficiency is the most prevalent nutritional deficiency, and creative means of delivering iron to high-risk groups need to be devised. An iron program (supplementation as fortification) should be considered when ...

■ *any group of adolescent girls is together in school or special classes.* Give them iron to build up their stores and compensate for menstrual blood losses.

■ *any group of women is together* (such as in a meeting at their farm co-op or well-baby clinic, in a health education session, literacy class, or loan solidarity group). Most women are anemic. They may not be willing to take iron during pregnancy so take advantage of all opportunities to give them iron.

■ *designing food aid programs that use processed food.* Flour, oil, condiments, and milk can be fortified with iron as well as iodine and vitamins.

■ *developing weaning foods.* Processed or fermented foods and germinated flours can be fortified with iron or can enhance iron absorption. Micronutrient-rich foods can be added to homemade porridges.

■ *designing horticultural projects.* Encourage the production and consumption of micronutrient-rich foods.

■ *designing social forestry projects.* Plant and animal sources of iron and vitamins A or C are abundant in multiuse forests.

■ *implementing livestock programs.* Use the programs to encourage household consumption of meat or animal by-products (especially of small stock) to make a major contribution to the daily intake of highly absorbed iron.

■ *improving pharmaceutical supply programs or essential drug programs.* Iron folate tablets are part of virtually every basic drug program yet they are almost always neglected by drug-system managers. Improvements in tablet color, coating, packaging, and distribution will make major contributions to improving compliance.

■ *designing any maternal-child health (MCH) program.* Iron deficiency is so prevalent in women and children that an MCH program that does not give high visibility to anemia control is seriously deficient.

■ *many children get transfusions for severe anemia.* Their need for additional iron, and perhaps for treatment of iron-depleting disease such as hookworm, is self-evident.

Successful national strategies address micronutrient malnutrition as a distinct problem and attack it through as many venues as possible: nutrition programs with specific micronutrient components, direct delivery of supplements to target populations, clinic-based programs to prevent and treat deficiencies during regularly scheduled visits, school interventions, agricultural policies with a nutritional focus, and food fortification (see Box 1.1 for an example of opportunities with a special emphasis on iron). Underlying these diverse efforts and essential to them is a simultaneous campaign to inform people about micronutrients and to guide consumers to incorporate them in their diet. Only such a campaign, using print media, advertising, counseling, and other means, can create conscious demand for nutritious food, which constitutes the fundamental resolution of the problem.

While the national strategy proceeds with the alleviation of poverty and the development of the health care system, specific micronutrient programs must be promoted. When the promotional efforts achieve a critical mass of agreement among political leaders and the public, an action program can begin on four planes at once, each with a progressively longer-term goal: (1) highly targeted, rapid interventions through the delivery of vitamin and mineral pills and other pharmaceuticals; (2) longer-term interventions through fortification of selected foods, if feasible; (3) consumer education programs to modify diets by building awareness of micronutrients; and (4) coordinated agricultural programs to increase the supply of micronutrient-rich food.

It is fortunate that the costs of these strategies are among the lowest of all health-related programs.

CHAPTER TWO

The Low Costs of Overcoming Vitamin and Mineral Deficiencies

W ITHIN an overall campaign of advocacy and education to create political support and popular demand for action on micronutrients, the three major ways of delivering micronutrients are:

1. *Supplementation* of the diet with pharmaceutical nutrients in capsule, tablet, injectable, or liquid
2. *Fortification* of food with nutrients
3. *Dietary change* by expanding the demand for, and supply of, nutrient-rich foods.

When considered separately or in any combination, these three modes involve low costs and high returns. The direct costs of delivering nutrients as supplements or in food are remarkably low. In Indonesia and the Philippines, it cost an estimated $0.25 per person (1984 dollars) to deliver vitamin A in capsules; in India in 1987, $0.05 per person to fortify salt with iodine; in Guatemala in 1980, $0.12 per person to fortify sugar with iron (Table 2.1).

Costs in terms of life-years free of illness (disability-adjusted life-year gained, or DALY) is a measure for comparing health interventions. Some of the lowest-cost interventions have per DALY cost ranges that vary from $2 to $10 (for tetanus immunization), to $15 to $75 (for fertility control) (Jamison 1993).[3]

Table 2.1   Costs of Micronutrient Control Programs

Micronutrient	Country/year	Estimated cost in US$/person (1994)	Estimated cost per person per year of protection (1994$)
Iodine			
Oil injection	Peru 1978	2.75	0.55
Oil injection	Zaire 1977	0.80	0.17
Oil injection	Indonesia 1986	1.25	0.25
Water fortification	Italy 1986	0.05	0.05
Salt fortification	India 1987	0.02–0.05	0.02–0.05
Vitamin A			
Sugar fortification	Guatemala 1976	0.17	0.17
Capsule	Haiti 1978	0.27–0.41	0.55–0.81
Capsule	Indonesia/Philippines 1975	0.25	0.50
Iron			
Salt fortification	India 1980	0.12	0.12
Sugar fortification	Guatemala 1980	0.12	0.12
Sugar fortification	1980	1.00	1.00
Tablets	1980	3.17–5.30	3.17–5.30

Source: Levin, Pollitt, Galloway, and McGuire 1993.

In these terms, micronutrient programs are extremely attractive: $4 per DALY for iron fortification, $8 for iodine fortification, and $29 for vitamin A fortification (Table 2.2). The most expensive strategy, supplementing the iodine intake of everyone under age 60, comes to $37 per DALY.

The costs of dietary change are less well documented than those of fortification and supplementation. One effective program in Nepal combined educating mothers in vitamin A nutrition with literacy based on a vitamin A–oriented curriculum; it cost $2 per person (the nutrition education alone cost about $1.25). Nutrition education about vitamin A prevented 1,085 deaths ($238 per death prevented) and 2,340 cases of xerophthalmia ($110 per case prevented) while nutrition education along with maternal literacy prevented 1,600 deaths ($252 per death prevented) and 3,510 cases of xerophthalmia ($115 per case prevented) (Tilden and others 1994). A project in Bangladesh to educate consumers about vitamin A and to stimulate production of foods containing it cost about $0.11 per person per year (not counting the $8 per person per year in vitamin A foods the family would need to consume).

These costs for dietary change seem much higher than those shown above for fortification and supplementation. But dietary change programs may be more sustainable at the family and community level when the sources of micronutrients are locally available—established behavior patterns don't depend on the regular resupply of promotional messages or of pharmaceuticals for effectiveness. Dietary change can also generate wider payoffs: a study of the Nepal program showed that greater maternal literacy and awareness of vitamin A generated other benefits in the area of child growth and the mother's use of health care (Tilden and others 1994). The greatest cost in these dietary change programs was that of the promoted foods, which were purchased by the family and often substituted for other foods in the family food basket.

Program Designs

With their finite budgets, developing countries must choose whether to aim their programs at specific subsets of the population (the poorest, pregnant women and preschool children, the already ill) or at the whole population,

Table 2.2   Returns on Nutrition Investments

Deficiency/remedy	Cost per life saved ($)	Discounted value ($) of productivity gained per program ($)	Cost per disability- adjusted life year gained
Iron deficiency			
Supplementation of pregnant women only	800	25	13
Fortification	2,000	84	4
Iodine deficiency			
Supplementation (repro-aged women only)	1,250	14	19
Supplementation (all people under 60)	4,650	6	37
Fortification	1,000	28	8
Vitamin A deficiency			
Supplementation (under 5 only)	325	22	9
Fortification	1,000	7	29
Nutrition education[a]	238	n.a.	n.a.
Nutrition education and maternal literacy[a]	252	n.a.	n.a.

n.a. Not applicable.
a. Tilden and others 1994.
Source: Levin, Pollitt, Galloway, and McGuire 1993. See Appendix B.

whether to develop nutritional self-sufficiency through dietary change or to focus on the rapid supply of nutrients through fortification and supplementation. The appropriate choices are not fixed for all places and times.

Examples of the trade-offs involved in various choices come from the Philippines and Indonesia. In the Philippines, investigators concluded that the ratio of costs to benefits was always lower for supplementation than for fortification or education (Popkin, Solon, Fernandez, and Latham 1980). In Indonesia investigators found that, at low annual micronutrient budget levels (less than $0.42 per person), dietary modification would be most cost-effective; at moderate levels ($0.43 to $0.87 per person), capsules would be preferred; and at higher levels, fortification was most cost-effective (Gross and Tilden 1988).

Supplementation and education, which require personal contact, can be relatively costly when targeted at those living in physically remote and culturally isolated regions. Theoretically, education generates new cultural norms for diet in these populations through their (presumably low-intensity) contact with the rest of the society. If this transmission happens at all, however, it does so only after a long and sustained period of change.

Because the success of fortification depends on the development of a product acceptable to the consumer and on the government's ability to enforce standards, its launch must be preceded by careful research, education, training, and institution building if it is not to risk failure. The scale of a fortification program is determined (1) by the foods to be fortified, and (2) by the proportion of the supply of those foods that is actually fortified. If a large part of the population is *not* at risk for a particular nutrient, one might want to select a food consumed by the needy and *only* by them. But if the cost of fortification is low—and in most cases it is—the extension to the non-needy may be administratively more practical and still economical.

Consider the case of salt, which is consumed by practically everyone. In almost every country in the world, adding iodine to refined salt would cost less than $0.10 per person per year. If the entire supply of salt were fortified and only half the population were at risk from iodine deficiency, the cost per needy person would double, but the amount would still be just $0.20 per person.

Successful fortification of a staple food may be one of the most equitable health interventions available—especially if the slight cost of the additional nutrients is absorbed by the government—because it reaches everyone, including the poor, pregnant women, and young children, populations that social services can never cover completely. Only the adequate enforcement of fortification standards (and a palatable product) will guarantee that the intended scale is actually achieved.

Public and Private Financing

Who should pay for micronutrient programs? Over the long run, programs that deliver micronutrients to those who can afford adequate caloric intake should be self-financing: with proper information, these consumers will have the knowledge and the access to the foodstuffs and supplements necessary to avoid nutritional deficiency without subsidy. And those who cannot afford adequate food should be receiving the needed nutrients from nutritional safety net programs, which are already being subsidized. Hence, ideally, no micronutrient program as such would be needed in the long term beyond efforts to sustain the population's knowledge regarding micronutrients.

In the short term, the lack of consumer awareness and the heavy social costs of malnutrition amply justify public intervention and subsidy to get countries with deficiencies on a nutritionally self-sufficient path. The specific strategy and financing plan for each country will be based on local diets, the structure of the food and drug industries, the coverage of public services, the sophistication of communications systems, and fiscal realities. Generally, assistance in the form of foreign exchange, price stabilization, and subsidies will be critical aspects of initial micronutrient programs.

Donor organizations and donor countries have a role in supplying the foreign exchange needed to support fortification and supplementation: for supplementation, pharmaceuticals will likely come from abroad; for fortification, the nutrients, the equipment to process the food, and the chemicals and laboratory equipment required for monitoring will also be largely of foreign origin.[4]

The synthetic nutrients used for fortification and supplementation are inexpensive, but the insecure food supply in many households and the substantial markup on the nutrients by commercial manufacturers can create the near-term need for subsidies and price controls. For example, vitamin A and iodine capsules cost under $0.50 per person per year as delivered; if they are sold through private retail outlets, however, some social marketing, surveillance, and price controls may be necessary to assure that the consumer is not being overcharged. Such markups can likewise lead to higher prices for fortified foods and the consequent shunning of them by consumers if the price is not subsidized. As all of the supplies of that food become fortified and awareness generates a preference for it, the need for price support dwindles.

The remainder of the costs—largely recurring costs of supplies, delivery, and monitoring—should be assumed partially by consumers and partially by the government. In most cases, for example, the consumer bears virtually all the costs of iodizing of salt, while the costs of regulatory enforcement are appropriately covered by the government. Although iodizing refined salt requires little additional cost (in the United States, iodized salt carries the same price as uniodized salt), iodizing crude salt requires more processing, extra drying, and new waterproof packaging, all contributing to higher cost to the consumer. Iodizing crude salt, then, presents another case for near-term subsidies, to be gradually phased out as the salt industry modernizes.

A Social, Not a Technical, Challenge

The tools to correct micronutrient malnutrition are well understood and technically easy to apply—supplementation, fortification, and dietary change through education and food diversification. The costs are low and the payoffs large. But designing a program on the basis of cost-effective technology does not determine the success of the program. A review of micronutrient programs around the world points to the creation of demand as the indispensable factor for success. Creating demand is a matter of modifying behaviors by easing resistance to dietary change—through education, demonstration, and advocacy—and by providing motivations to seek such change. Leaders must be motivated to support nutrition programs; beyond them, health care workers, teachers, the business community, mothers, and consumers at large must demand the supplements, nutrient-rich foods, and fortified foods that deliver good nutrition.

Such popular demand, which creates political support, is essential to the sustainability of micronutrient programs. Therefore a consumer perspective should be included in all elements of micronutrient programs, including supplementation, fortification, agricultural initiatives, and communications. As demand is generated, supply must also be guaranteed through improved program management.

CHAPTER THREE

The Delivery of Supplements

PHARMACEUTICAL supplementation can appear to be an easy solution to the micronutrient problem. In fact, supplementation is as complex as any other approach, if not more so: it requires a good logistical system capable of delivering high-quality pharmaceuticals when and where they are needed and a good social marketing program to sensitize and inform the population about micronutrients. But these elements only prepare the ground, so to speak, and set the stage for the effective delivery of micronutrients. The actual uptake of supplements by the targeted populations requires trained, motivated health care workers who can communicate effectively with consumers to overcome their fears, misinformation, and ignorance.

Training and Support of Health Care Workers

Taking pills and getting injections may require deep changes in behavior and belief. The neediest populations often see the nutritional quality of their diet as irrelevant to fatigue or other forms of ill health. Fears also play a part: for example, a common fear among women is that an iron pill or iodized oil injection is a contraceptive. For pregnant women, taking iron means maintaining a new daily behavior that (1) may not be pleasant given the fishy aftertaste of iron and the constipation it may induce, and (2) may seem pointless after the women experience rapid relief from symptoms (even if the underlying anemia lingers on). Thus, for targeted populations—and for mothers in particular, who must obtain supplements frequently, sometimes daily—merely showing up for the injection or actually taking the pill or giving it to a child often implies a great accomplishment: perceiving the three-way connection between health, the *ongoing* need for nutrients, and the supplement.

In supplementation, therefore, much rides on the abilities and commitment of health providers. They must know enough and be sensitive enough to explain the nature and importance of the capsules, pills, or injectables; to determine which family members need them and in what dosage and frequency; to tell when and where to get them; and to both warn and reassure the consumer about the supplement's possible side effects.

In addition, the delivery of pharmaceuticals often requires health care workers to make strategic choices that must be informed by their knowledge of the particular attitudes and life situations of the targeted population. A campaign of supplementation can be far more effective when it includes consumers in the planning phase to learn the attitudes and perceptions of the targeted populations.

Minimizing Supply Problems

An effective social marketing campaign, combined with the effective counseling of consumers by health care workers, has a two-way benefit. It helps increase the acceptability and penetration of the supplementation campaign, and it helps create a public demand for, and expectation of, good nutrition. The acceptance of supplementation is a necessary but insufficient condition for a long-term program; unless consumers *demand* supplementation out of a sense of *entitlement*, health providers are more likely to forget to distribute the nutrients, the supplies are more likely to be given to the non-needy or deteriorate in warehouses, and the program is much more likely to fail, initial successes notwithstanding.

Indeed, many supply problems, which the SCN[5] has found to be more important than client noncompliance as a cause of iron program failures, are rooted in a lack of worker training and client education. One East African country, for example, almost dropped vitamin A from its list of essential drugs because health workers didn't know when to prescribe it and the community didn't demand it. Administrators saw the product accumulate in storage and thought it wasn't needed; training and community education remedied the problem. Training also permits workers to anticipate and accommodate increased demand for supplements from newly informed consumers and to direct scarce supplies of supplements to the neediest.

Supplementation Programs

To boost coverage levels rapidly, one Southeast Asian country in 1980 introduced a vertical (that is, single-focus) program (alongside its existing health care program) to deliver vitamin A supplements in schools, community centers, and other locales of convenience and opportunity. After two years, coverage had increased from 6 to 77 percent (West and Sommer 1987), a high rate, although the populations missed by the program were probably the neediest. Today, however, coverage has fallen below 50 percent because momentum could not be sustained. If coverage dwindles in a high-intensity, initially successful program like this one, then normal programs are not likely to sustain themselves.

In a South Asian country, a "universal" program of vitamin A supplementation, which uses existing health care providers, reaches only about 36 percent of the population (probably the least vulnerable portion) largely because the public health care system has poor coverage. Furthermore, coverage has fallen over time, perhaps because of worker apathy or because the intended beneficiaries do not perceive the need for vitamin A or the threat of blindness from vitamin A deficiency. If the intended beneficiaries were actively seeking the supplements, coverage would not be so low or decline over time, yet rarely do supplementation programs include any social marketing.

In general, social marketing to raise demand and lend the program urgency, more aggressive targeting of populations, increased outreach, and improved quality of services are needed to raise and sustain the coverage of supplementation programs (see Box 3.1).

Targeting Special Groups and Using Existing Outreach Programs

Targeting is a critical issue in the design of a micronutrient supplementation program because the deficiencies may affect specific subgroups in the population. Even in countries considered to have endemic vitamin A deficiency (Bangladesh, India, Indonesia), the prevalence of signs of moderate deficiency (night blindness) rarely exceeds 5 percent in young children (in Bangladesh 2.6 percent of preschoolers were night-blind in 1991). With iodine deficiency, an incidence of visible goiter in 20 percent or more of the population is a sign of a serious public health problem. Iron deficiency commonly affects 30 percent of the general population and as much as 75 percent of pregnant women. Targeting is economically desirable if it can be done at low cost. In the case of iron, the deficiency may be so prevalent that presumptive treatment of all pregnant or reproductive-aged women may be more cost-effective than a program of

BOX 3.1 LESSONS LEARNED FROM SUPPLEMENTATION PROGRAMS

■ Educate community leaders to win them as allies.

■ Rank target groups and try to reach highest priority groups first.

■ Induce families to come to clinics by marketing the supplement as health-promoting rather than as a prevention for blindness or cretinism— these diseases are sufficiently rare that people will think they won't be affected.

■ Extend the program beyond the clinics—the Expanded Program on Immunization can be useful.

■ Deliver supplies on time and in the right amounts.

■ Make sure health care providers know exactly what to do and why— train and supervise for performance.

■ Schedule regular weeks or months for supplements to ease management and marketing problems.

■ Distribute supplementation records to beneficiaries and check supplementation status whenever a target-group member appears at a clinic.

■ Counsel household decision-makers about giving micronutrient-rich foods to young children and pregnant and lactating women. This includes breastfeeding promotion.

■ Integrate pharmaceutical supplementation with the development of longer-term solutions.

---

screening plus therapeutic treatment. In general the options for targeting are as follows:

1. *Universal targeting, or nontargeting* (targeting vitamin A to all preschool children; targeting iron folate tablets to all pregnant women; targeting iodized oil to all women of reproductive age; or all schoolchildren). In practice, universal targeting means reaching the most willing and accessible population.

2. *Medical targeting.* This includes targeting vitamin A to children with xerophthalmia, chronic diarrhea, severe acute respiratory infections, growth failure, tuberculosis, or measles; and targeting iron to premature and low-birthweight babies.

3. *Geographic or seasonal targeting.* Iodized oil is usually targeted to high-altitude areas and places beyond the reach of commercial salt markets. Vitamin A supplements may be required only during the dry season or in semiarid areas. Iron may be targeted to malarious or hookworm-infected regions.

4. *Targeting using biochemical tests.* This is generally inefficient and uneconomical except where prevalence of deficiency is very low or danger of toxic overdose very high.

Medical targeting of vitamin A works well because ill children are likely to be brought to a health center, which facilitates distribution. Determining the coverage of such programs is difficult, however, because the total population of sick children is variable and unknown. Outreach is also difficult in this situation because health workers are unlikely to know when a child falls ill. Nonetheless, medical targeting can be an economical means of getting vitamin A to a subpopulation of children who need it badly.

If universal distribution is the mode of choice, the Expanded Program on Immunization (EPI) can help deliver supplements to remote areas (see Box 3.2). Many countries with the EPI immunize 80 percent or more of the EPI target group of 6- to 14-week-old children. Using the EPI village visits and programs to deliver micronutrient supplements to all children, as well as to adults, would yield a major advance in coverage of micronutrient supplements.

EPI campaigns as currently configured are better suited to oral iodine (which needs only one annual dose) than to vitamin A (which needs to be given every four to six months) because national campaign days usually run for two days

---

BOX 3.2 SUPPLEMENTATION THROUGH THE EXPANDED PROGRAM ON IMMUNIZATION

It will take a long time for iodized salt to address iodine deficiency in the remote districts of Nepal, so the country has set up a free-standing program to supply iodized oil to those regions through the infrastructure of the Expanded Program on Immunization (EPI).

The goal is universal coverage in a phased succession of districts, with repeated administration of injected iodized oil after three to five years. Workers focus community participation on mobilizing interest in iodine deficiency and the uptake of iodized oil. The poor infrastructure and remoteness of the mountainous areas, which limit access to iodized salt, also make laboratory-based surveillance of treatment progress impossible. Coverage and impact figures are not available, but through limited epidemiological assessments of goiter and cretinism and through other indicators such as the disappearance of stocks, the program is seen as a success.

The director of the program credits the success to many of the same factors associated with the success of EPI and malaria control, namely, clearly delineated objectives and targets, "clarity of purpose," a core group of supervisory and managerial level workers with experience in surveys and program management under difficult conditions, and a campaign mentality (Acharya 1991).

four to six weeks apart. With some expansion of responsibilities and target groups, however, EPI workers could be used to deliver vitamin A every four to six months or during specific months. In countries with highly seasonal deficiencies (Nepal is an example), a single dose, properly timed, could be adequate. But in many countries, vitamin A deficiency is a year-round problem. Iron tonic could be delivered through EPI to children above 6 months of age but it has not yet been tried.

Where vitamin A and iodine deficiencies are geographically, ethnically, or socioeconomically concentrated, targeted rather than national programs may be preferable (although emerging evidence on the effects of subclinical deficiencies suggests that broader rather than narrow targeting may be warranted). High-risk areas are fairly easy to delineate on the basis of low iodine content in soils and water or of goiter incidence in school children. These high-risk areas often coincide with high altitude or flood plains because the iodine has been leached away over millennia. Vitamin A clusters less well geographically than iodine, although it is likely to occur in arid areas. Although the risk of vitamin A deficiency may correlate with season or with rainfall levels, this indicator is not specific enough for general application. Epidemiological or dietary data on vitamin A deficiency is likely to be needed.

India seeks delivery of vitamin A to young children through a two-track approach involving both the health system and the Integrated Child Development Services (ICDS) program. The health system, through the national immunization program, gives vitamin A supplements to children under 1 year of age. Older preschool children receive vitamin A supplementation twice yearly from health workers, of whom there are about one for every three villages. In addition, through about 250,000 workers based in about half of India's villages, ICDS administers vitamin A—on demand where supplies are stable and otherwise twice yearly—to children under 6 years of age. Midwives and, increasingly, ICDS workers are also being enlisted to provide megadoses of vitamin A to women immediately after childbirth, thereby reaching not only the women but, through their breast milk, the babies.

Other potential avenues of increased coverage could be school personnel, agricultural extension agents, religious leaders, and private pharmacists. In a Muslim country, for instance, iodine capsules could be distributed annually at local mosques on Eid, the celebration ending Ramadan.

Supplements could also be supplied through retail stores (free, at-cost, or in exchange for a coupon from the health center) where public drug management is not adequate. (The approach has had some success in contraceptive social marketing.) In one African country, the private pharmacies are used to deliver iron tablets prescribed at the health clinic. In light of the popularity of pseudonutrients—ineffective, falsely advertised, and potentially dangerous concoctions often sought out even in traditional cultures to cure disease—and of vitamin supplements of dubious value (especially injections of vitamin B complex), health workers must carefully inform consumers about the kind of supplement to take, the dosage, who is to take it and when, and the dangers of overdosing. In general, the production, advertising, and packaging of privately marketed micronutrient supplements needs tight regulation coupled with consumer education to prevent fraud and assure quality control.

Biomedical screening can also guide targeting. The medical preference is to screen clients before prescribing therapeutic treatment. In large-scale national micronutrient programs, however, the cost of screening can exceed the cost of treatment. Where the prevalence of a deficiency is high enough to be a public health problem by World Health Organization (WHO) criteria, then presumptive treatment may be preferred. This is particularly true of iron supplementation for pregnant women. Toxicity becomes a potential problem with supplements when the population becomes more sufficient in the nutrient.[6] In that case, community screening may be adequate—a subsample of people are selected, and if the prevalence of the deficiency is high, all target-age individuals receive supplements.

CHAPTER FOUR

Successful Fortification

As with supplementation, fortification has the appeal of a panacea: if the right food is selected, high coverage of the population is assured. Indeed, fortification—the addition of specific vitamins and minerals to foods and water—has eradicated most vitamin and mineral deficiencies in the industrial countries (see Box 4.1). Unfortunately, an ideal food vehicle for fortification is not available in every situation. Nonetheless many foods have successfully been fortified in a number of countries (Table 4.1), and with dietary habits changing rapidly and food industries becoming more sophisticated, fortification is likely to be feasible in the near future in most countries.

BOX 4.1 HOW FORTIFICATION WON THE WEST

Dietary diversification and poverty alleviation have eradicated many historic nutritional deficiencies—pellagra, scurvy, rickets, and beriberi among them—but by far the most direct *policy* intervention in the West has been food fortification. Fortification of margarine with vitamin D is thought to have eliminated rickets from Britain and Northern Europe in the early part of this century. Fortification of refined flour with iron in the United States and Sweden is credited with the dramatic reduction of anemia. The introduction of iodized salt in Switzerland in 1929 spelled the end of cretinism in that country.

Table 4.1   Foods Successfully Used for Fortification

Micronutrient	Vehicle
Iodine	Salt
	Bread
	Water
Iron	Wheat flour and bakery products
	Cornmeal
	Rice
	Salt
	Sugar
	Condiments
	Milk
	Infant cereals
	Processed foods
Vitamin A	Sugar
	Cooking fat
	Margarine
	Vegetable oils
	MSG
	Tea

Source: Venkatesh Mannar 1993.

Problems with Voluntary Fortification

Over the long term, micronutrient deficiencies can be largely corrected through fortification at a cost per capita that is affordable by most of the intended beneficiaries. But fortification generally is not carried out voluntarily by the private food processing sector. Voluntary fortification has worked well in the United States for salt and flour and in the Netherlands for bread, because fortification is high on the list of consumer food preferences in these countries.

In most developing countries, however, consumer demand is lacking, and voluntary fortification is unlikely to work because those companies that act first to fortify take more risks than those that act later or never act at all. For example, the costs of product development, market research, and advertising will be borne by the first company to fortify its product. Initially, either the price of the pioneering product will be higher than that of its competitors, at the cost of market share, or the profits of the pioneering company will be cut. On the one hand, competitors that add fortification later will get a free ride from the pioneering company, which may not be able to recoup profits or market share, as the case may be. On the other hand, successful marketing could reap profits for the first company to introduce fortified food.

Consumer demand for nutritious food—natural or fortified—is the key to the long-term success of all micronutrient programs, including fortification. Because such awareness and demand does not exist to a sufficient degree in most developing countries, the government may need to take the lead and require fortification of strategic products. The two most important determinants of early success in fortification programs are the selection of the right foods to fortify and the level of industry compliance with fortification rules.

Whether the food chosen is the "right" one is largely a matter of consumer acceptance. In the past, fortification advocates have sought a single food for fortification, but under some conditions it may be more effective to select several food vehicles in order to reach segments of the population that have different diets (see Box 4.2).

In general, fortification is considered a universal program, but targeted fortification may sometimes be appropriate. In Guatemala, the school-feeding program uses a biscuit fortified with a number of vitamins and minerals. The biscuits are baked by local bakeries and the vitamin-mineral premix is distributed to them by the government. Undoubtedly the children in schools are a self-selected, relatively privileged group but they are easy to reach, and they profit educationally from the added nutrition. In South Africa, the Asian community was found to be the only subpopulation that was deficient in iron, so curry powder was fortified with iron. In Chile and the United States, infant foods are fortified with iron because that is one of the most vulnerable groups. One could also target foods consumed primarily by the poor or distributed in welfare programs.

The Importance of Consumer Participation and Education

Fortified foods must be extensively tested in the development phase to ensure the feasibility of manufacture and their acceptability to the consumer. Such testing, covering availability, price, taste, appearance, and similarity to the unfortified product, is critical to ensure that the fortified food will not meet significant consumer resistance. If fortified products are even slightly off color, for example, they may be unacceptable to consumers.

Fortification programs must include an educational component to motivate the consumer to purchase what otherwise might seem to be an unknown product that might be in direct competition with the old. Although technical manipulations are supposed to minimize the detectable difference between fortified and unfortified foods, consumers may consider the fortificant to be

BOX 4.2 LESSONS OF EXPERIENCE FROM FORTIFICATION PROGRAMS

■ Consumer education—about the nature of vitamin and mineral deficiencies, their cost, and the benefits of fortified food—is essential.

■ Intake of the nutrient must be well below estimated requirements.

■ The food to be fortified must be chosen carefully:

1. It must be a staple of the target population to assure uptake of the fortificant (and to ensure that demand will not fall under the price increases required to pay for fortification).

2. It must retain its desirability (color, flavor, texture, cooking properties) after fortification.

3. Feasibility studies must show that its fortification will be fairly easy

and inexpensive, or research must develop such methods.

4. The fortification sites must be easily monitored.

■ The law must require that all supplies of the staple, domestic and imported, be fortified.

■ Duties and fees on imported fortificants should be waived.

■ The staff for monitoring compliance with fortification must be large enough for the task, well trained, and motivated to do an honest and thorough job.

■ Producers must receive incentives such as technical assistance, subsidization for small producers, and journalistic coverage of good performers, as well as face sanctions such as swift but not overly punitive punishment of offenders and journalistic exposés of noncompliant companies.

unnatural or "chemical"—witness the resistance to fluoridation of water in the United States.

When fortified foods cost more than the unfortified, consumer demand needs to be oriented toward the fortified product. Well-tested marketing techniques can be used to get consumers to try a new product. The results of consumer tests must be given continually to public and private decisionmakers so they are informed when their support is needed. A way around some of these difficulties—but not around the fundamental need to gain the general support of consumers—is to require fortification of *all* stocks of a selected foodstuff, especially if it is a staple. In the case of salt, for example, all salt for human and animal consumption should be iodized to prevent any "leakage" of unfortified stocks into the food system.

Universal and Mandatory Fortification

Health ministers in many countries are not able or willing to control and motivate private industry. In such cases, a specified set of responsibilities and
actions regarding fortification should be passed on to the ministry of industry.[7]
The preferred regulatory option requires fortification and yet also gives indus-

---

**BOX 4.3   INDIA FORTIFIES SALT
THROUGH TRANSPORT CONTROLS**

Salt iodization is well on its way to
becoming universal in India, largely
because of government controls on
rail transport. In 1984 the Indian Par-
liament required the universal
iodization of salt, giving to states the
responsibility of enforcement. All
states (except the four southern states
and Maharashtra, which have no
widespread iodine deficiency) subsequently banned the importation, production, and trade in uniodized salt.
The fines, however, are not punitive
enough to induce compliance. The
public subsidization of potassium iodate between 1987 and 1992 was an
effective incentive to industry to iodate
their salt, but the subsidy ceased in
1992 because of budgetary pressure.

Salt producers comply because of
the control afforded by the geography
of salt markets. Salt is produced in
western and southern India and must
travel by rail to the consumer markets
elsewhere in the country. Rail car allotments are scarce and sold only by
the full trainload. They are worth a
great deal to traders. The government
permits salt producers to use 2,000-
ton, full train allotments only if the salt
is iodized. The Salt Department in the
Ministry of Industry monitors the
iodization of salt and certifies the salt
for shipment. This system also allows
India to avoid the common problem of
inducing small producers to comply;
such producers generally sell to salt
traders who have the capacity and the
equipment to iodize their salt. By controlling the transport of salt, the government can thus effectively demand
iodization.

Not all is solved, however. Today,
3 million tons of salt are iodized out of
total salt consumption of 4.5 million
tons. One of the problems is that the
lumpy brown "rock" salt preferred in
some parts of the country is only
coated with iodine. The consumer
washes off the iodine when he or she
washes the salt (which is customary
for the brown salt). Consumer education is needed either to channel demand toward the whiter iodized salt
(where the iodine is integrated into
the structure of the salt) or to discourage the washing of the salt. In addition, a bureaucratic problem is the
Salt Commissioner's lack of fiscal
authority over the health inspectors,
which causes needless delays and
inefficiencies.

---

try persuasive incentives to adopt the regulations. Such incentives can include low-interest loans to purchase new fortification equipment, reduced tariffs and duties on fortificants, technical assistance, import subsidies, and special certification or labeling provisions. In India, producers of iodized salt get preferential rail car allotments (see Box 4.3) to move salt from production centers to markets across the country. Government enterprises that control most of the market for a specific food can adopt fortification and thereby push private-sector companies to do the same (if consumer reaction is correctly gauged and accounted for).[8]

One approach to mandatory fortification is to have a national bureau of standards or the ministry of industry and trade establish a "standard of identity" for the product that specifies the level of fortification in establishing licensing regulations. Another way is to establish regulations for fortifying specific foods through the food control laws. Legislation, which could take several years to be approved, should not establish technical details but should instead empower the appropriate ministry or department (usually health, or agriculture, or industry) to regulate fortification of appropriate foods at levels that will ensure effectiveness and at the same time be safe. Using these powers, the ministry can then issue directives or regulations fixing standards and specification for enforcement. Choice between a fortified and unfortified product may need to be eliminated for both producers and consumers.

Experience has shown that the most successful fortification programs have been mandatory.[9] Attempts to require fortification only in certain regions has not worked. Some countries, for example, have attempted to iodize salt only in the regions where endemic iodine deficiency exists. Because markets in most food products do not follow political boundaries or coincide with epidemiological patterns, this differential application of mandatory fortification is not effective. It burdens regional producers unfairly and provides further opportunities for profiteering.[10]

Ensuring industry compliance with fortification programs requires an understanding of how private industry functions for a specific food in a specific country. This will determine both the incentives and the legal sanctions needed, price and cost factors, technical assistance and capital requirements, and public-private responsibilities.

CHAPTER FIVE

Dietary Change through Education and Policy

CONSUMERS can improve the nutritional quality of their diets if they are guided by well-designed communications and have ready access to micronutrient-rich foods that are affordable and acceptable.

Educating Consumers

Consumers must believe that the desired change in their dietary behavior will bring tangible benefits. Vitamin A programs in four Asian countries could not persuade mothers to give green, leafy vegetables to their young children to avoid blindness, a malady too rare to compel a change in behavior. The promotion of good health, however, and the elevation of vitamin A foods from being merely "useful" to "essential," produced substantial results.

The nutrition message is most effective when it reaches consumers through many channels, including the mass media reinforced by personal contacts at locations such as schools, the workplace, and health clinics. Some programs have used a great variety of vehicles to carry the desired message: plastic produce bags, stickers, mobile drama groups, singers, comic books, recipe contests, and quiz shows. Spokespeople in advertising campaigns should be both attractive and credible; physicians and entertainers who can believably deliver a health message can be effective in such a role.

These educational efforts should stimulate the demand for more nutritious food in the diet, and they can also stimulate needed support for programs to expand the supply of such food (see Box 5.1).

The Influence of Agricultural Policies

Regarding cultivated foods, agricultural policies can send some powerful signals to farmers to encourage (or discourage) certain crops.[11] Agriculture research

---

BOX 5.1   STEPS TOWARD RAISING MICRONUTRIENT LEVELS IN THE FOOD SUPPLY

■ *Survey the food system.* A survey should reveal what foods contribute to the year-round supply of micronutrients and are being consumed by the target groups, whether gardening and/or gathering foods is a tradition, what foods are sold, and whether the additional income is used to buy other foods high in the micronutrients.

■ *Determine the demand for garden foods and gathered foods relative to their supply.* Learn whether women have time for additional food production or collecting or whether other groups, like men and the elderly, could be targeted to help increase the family's supply of micronutrient-rich foods. If traditional beliefs about certain foods cannot be changed, look for alternative sources of the desired micronutrient that do not violate traditions and taboos.

■ *Assess the nutrition status of target groups and develop a monitoring system to show nutritional impact of gardening interventions.* Set precise targets for consumption levels of micronutrient-rich foods that are adequate for different ages of children and women.

■ *Identify agriculture extension workers, successful local gardeners, and other people in the community who can give technical assistance in gardening or gathering wild foods.* Training these people to improve horticultural techniques would help improve chances of success.

■ *Study local markets to determine whether home production of certain foods might disrupt marketing and later discourage production.* There is much controversy about selling produce from gardens because the income often does not benefit vulnerable groups, hence the need for a strong nutrition education and social marketing program so that families reserve at least part of the food they grow for themselves or so that the income generated from gardens is used to buy other micronutrient-rich foods.

■ *Include beneficiaries in the planning, implementation, monitoring, and evaluation of the program.* Local leaders should assume responsibility for identifying demand for the program and the types of interventions most useful to beneficiaries.

and extension can make particular crops more profitable or feasible to cultivate. Recent evidence suggests that selective breeding, seed treatment, and
mineral fertilization can improve the micronutrient content of grains. In Thailand, agriculture extension agents distributed ivy gourd plants—which had
been identified as a key vitamin A food—and advised farmers on its cultivation. When the so-called "disease-resistant" crop developed insect and
mold problems, scientists in collaboration with traditional experts solved the
problem.

Policies usually favor only those horticultural products and field and tree
crops that sell well in export markets or otherwise have good effects on employment and income. But these foods may offer little to improve local nutrition. For example, in many countries, narrow policies to promote either food
grains or export crops have reduced substantially the production of legumes,
generally a good source of both protein and iron (Figure 5.1).

Policy Support for Subsistence Horticulture

An important new area for agricultural policy is the encouragement of subsis-
tence horticulture. For policymakers and extension agents, food grown for

Figure 5.1   World per Capita Availability of Legumes

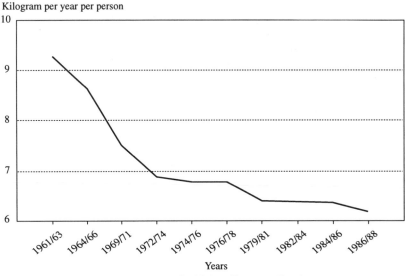

Kilogram per year per person

Source: FAO 1992 database (AGROSTAT/PC, Food Balance Sheets, FAO, Rome).

home consumption does not have the status of marketed crops. Further reducing the status of home gardens is the fact that they are usually considered to be the women's domain and that they are cultivated in more traditional ways. Home gardens can, however, be both a major household food resource and a source of income, and much more could be done to elevate their status and productivity. The Asian Vegetable Research and Development Center, in Taiwan (affiliated with the Consultative Group on International Agricultural Research, CGIAR) has developed several garden designs that serve nutritional purposes as well as generate income.

Horticultural products generally require copious amounts of water and are highly perishable. Public policy can greatly assist in the expansion by supporting the improvement of water systems, helping create more marketing outlets, improving roads and storage facilities to reduce farm-to-market spoilage, and advancing preservation techniques. Proper food preservation is particularly important for vitamin A, which is often highly seasonal in its availability.[12]

Preserving Foraged Foods

With foraged crops, the key policy issues relate more to land use and preservation of natural resources than to active cultivation. Forest land, meadows, wetlands, fallow land, and even weeds in cultivated fields have traditionally supplied much of the variety (and micronutrients) in people's diets. Many of these foods are unavailable in markets. The destruction of forests can seriously limit the access of people living nearby to meat, edible leaves, and fruit. From both an environmental and nutritional standpoint, preserving these lands in the wild state or encouraging nearby communities to husband them wisely is highly desirable.[13]

In general, food policies can support a diversified food base if they give due weight to dietary quality; push the development of varied sources of nutritious food, including home gardens; protect foraging areas; and actively work against negative trends in the quality of the food supply.

CHAPTER SIX

Characteristics of Successful Micronutrient Programs

ACTION in every country must start with a situation analysis to determine the nature and magnitude of the problem and the adequacy of current policies and programs. Many countries have performed these analyses as Children's Summit action plans through UNICEF or in preparation for the annual International Conference on Nutrition. The initial analysis stage is crucial to establishing local "ownership" of the program—a commitment to it on the part of experts and leaders. In Tanzania, for instance, national ownership resulted from a deliberate effort to have national professionals do their own problem assessment. Generally such assessments are made on the basis of outdated, unrepresentative, and inadequate data, but the quality of the data matters less than the motivation it generates. External consultants may be needed, but local control of the program is desirable for its long-range vitality.

Situation Analysis

Situation analysis must often be based on best guesses from scanty data. Rather than wait for nationally representative epidemiological data to justify action, the project should use "good enough" evidence initially; it should be prepared to adapt to new findings, and it should include information systems that will improve future assessments.

The "situation" in a situation analysis is more than an estimate of the prevalence of malnutrition. It also includes important dietary and behavioral factors as well as relevant interactions of deficiencies and disease (for instance, the coexistence of malaria and hookworm) that contribute to micronutrient malnutrition. The analysis should assess the coverage, quality, and cost of current efforts to remedy the problem, and it should also evaluate resources that could be marshaled in the future, including key food industries and markets.

The initial program design, as well as the initial analysis, must allow for modification; a detailed blueprint for short-term and long-term phases of a program is bound to run afoul of reality. Experience suggests that flexible program design complemented by interim evaluation, appropriate information systems, and consultation with intended beneficiaries helps generate effective and sustainable programs. Equally clear is the fact that programs require national political support and long-term commitment. Under most circumstances, external technical and financial assistance is needed as well.

In Thailand, the general direction of the program was established at the outset—addressing vitamin A deficiency through dietary means—but the strategy was developed as the program evolved and intended beneficiaries participated in it. In this iterative fashion, the beneficiaries and program staff identified the key food for promotion, the means of promoting it, the most persuasive messages, and ways of increasing the availability of vitamin A foods. This last issue led them into agricultural promotion and extension.

One characteristic of all successful country cases is the use of pilot projects and feasibility studies to try out delivery systems, communications concepts, or alternative sources of micronutrients. This experimentation, when combined with national advocacy and leadership, has led to revisions in program design that were not anticipated initially (for example, the use of agricultural extension). Information systems have facilitated further improvements as programs have been implemented.

Setting Priorities

After completion of the situation analysis comes the need to set priorities among nutrients and intervention options. In Tanzania, for example, program leaders decided that iodine was the simplest, and therefore the first, deficiency to attack, doing so with both supplementation via iodized oil capsules and iodine-fortified salt. Once the control of iodine deficiencies was well established, the government traded on the goodwill generated by that effort and moved on to tackle vitamin A deficiency, this time through supplementation via capsules plus promotion of the production and consumption of fruits and vegetables rich in vitamin A. Tanzania addressed the correction of iron deficiency last, and that component is the least advanced.

In contrast, one East Asian country tackled vitamin A deficiency first because advocacy by scientists and nongovernmental organizations (NGOs), plus dramatic results from a pilot project that used supplements, made it a "high profile" problem with political support for a resolution.

Unfortunately, supplementation with vitamin A capsules has been this country's major micronutrient strategy for almost twenty years. It has not developed longer-term vitamin A strategies, such as nutrition education and the promotion of home gardens, with anything but a minor emphasis, nor has it moved on to raise awareness and develop solutions to iodine and iron deficiencies.[14]

Short-term Supplementation Goals as Part of a Long-term Dietary Improvement Strategy

Micronutrient programs require a long-term vision right from the start, even if it initially concentrates on supplementation. A long-term vision means legitimizing food sources of micronutrients in advocacy and educational materials, developing plans for fortification to be phased in over time (if appropriate), and simultaneously promoting consumption of micronutrient-rich foods.

Overreliance on vitamin A capsules in one South Asian country caused consumers as well as health care workers to view supplementation as the only legitimate micronutrition strategy; phasing in dietary solutions is now proving very difficult. In an East African country, by contrast, because supplementation is seen as therapeutic—vitamin A capsules for sick children and iron tablets for pregnant women—food sources are seen as the essential preventive strategy.

The Importance of Feedback to Program Evolution

Feedback from a program during its implementation is critical to its flexibility and its ability to evolve. The information systems should be as simple as possible.

Programs that use nationally representative data to log progress and calculate social costs of deficiencies should use them sparingly because they consume time, resources, and personnel. The WHO classification of deficient countries provides an adequate basis for taking action. Where national surveys are not available, other sources of information should be exploited. Rapid assessment techniques or collection of relevant information in the process of program design and implementation can accomplish both the statistical and programmatic tasks.

Program designers should choose deficiency indicators with regard to the practical realities of data collection and with due respect to people's fears and time constraints.[15] Proxy measures of deficiencies (interviews about night blindness or breathlessness from exertion) and data from neighboring countries can be used. Perhaps more important than assessment of the micronutrient status of a population is monitoring the progress of program implementation. In fortification programs this means sampling the fortified food at the food plant and at the retail level. Some countries also test salt supplies in transit at police checkpoints. Others test the food at the household level. With the new generation of inexpensive, pocket-sized assessment kits, a food inspector or even a concerned consumer can check food for iodine and iron.

Monitoring supplementation programs involves tracking flows of supplements from the central warehouse to the periphery and ultimately to the consumer. Uptake rates are a good indicator for iodine and vitamin A coverage, but monitoring the distribution of iron requires some indicator of compliance—women's reports or disappearance of the tablets. Focus groups can also help overcome compliance problems.[16]

Monitoring dietary change programs requires discussions with intended beneficiaries on eating and feeding behaviors. It might also be possible to monitor price, availability, or sales volume of specific foods. (See Box 6.1.)

Sustainability

Political commitment is a key to getting funding for new programs and to keep getting them funded. Yet political support alone is unlikely to sustain a program long enough to outlive the micronutrient problem, and popular support must be generated. A politically powerful aspect of micronutrient programs is that people often feel better fast and the incidence of terrible disabilities is quickly reduced. Because these outcomes can be attributed unambiguously to the micronutrient programs themselves, the political leadership can take the credit for improved well-being. In Tanzania, for example, the renewed sense of vigor after iodine supplementation, especially when communicated directly to the nation's president, was effective feedback in support of the program. Thus, advocacy is best when grounded on both the impact of deficiencies and the effectiveness of interventions.

Low cost and high cost-effectiveness also enhance sustainability. If a government cannot afford to carry on a program after donors withdraw, it isn't viable. Cost and cost-effectiveness should be priority considerations in setting national strategies. One aspect of economic sustainability relates to the foreign exchange costs of an intervention. To the extent that interventions rely on imported materials (especially supplements and fortificants), a program may be

BOX 6.1 APPROPRIATE MONITORING

In Ecuador, limited resources did not permit sampling or laboratory analysis of the entire population for uptake of iodine through salt. Instead, social and epidemiological research enabled the program to undertake low cost, probabilistic monitoring in high risk communities.

■ In large communities (more than 120 children in school), because more than 80 percent of families use iodized salt, only smaller communities are monitored.

■ In smaller villages, teachers ask students what kind of salt they use at home (iodine deficiency is concentrated in families that do not use iodized salt). Iodized salt is very white and comes in small plastic packages; because uniodized salt is grainy and yellow and is not packaged, students can easily point to their family's salt.

■ If more than half of families use iodized salt, the community was considered low risk.

■ If half or less of the families use iodized salt, a medical team carries out a thyroid assessment and obtains urine samples from at least thirty children for iodine analysis. A concentration of iodine above a specified level classifies the community as medium risk; a concentration below that level defines high risk.

■ All high-risk individuals under the age of 45 are injected with iodized oil.

■ One hundred sentinel posts were established for ongoing surveillance using goiter assessment and urinary iodine.

---

unsustainable during periods of economic crisis when foreign exchange is scarce. Dietary change becomes a more appealing approach under these conditions, particularly where the exchange rate is overvalued.

Technical sustainability is also important. Not only must an intervention be technically efficient to be cost-effective, it also must be appropriate for the institutional capacity of the implementing agency. Moreover, the technology must be adaptable to changing environments (both institutional and epidemiological). Water fortification with iodine, for example, may start as a basic, household-level technology—adding drops of tincture of iodine to the family water pot. As hand pumps become available, the technology may need to change to community-level fortification by putting iodine-impregnated modules in pumps (see Box 6.2). In several more years, the technology may need to change again as centralized water systems are installed, facilitating water iodization at the water treatment plant. Or perhaps salt iodization would replace

BOX 6.2 APPROPRIATE TECHNOLOGY

Well water and pump water can now be easily fortified with iodine for a year at a time with a plastic cylinder developed by Rhône Poulenc Foundation. The cylinder, which contains an iodine-infused polymer, is inserted directly into the water and slowly releases iodine sufficient to meet the needs of 1,500 people for one year. The cylinder needs to be changed annually. In Mali, a one-year test reduced moderate to severe iodine deficiency (as measured by urinary iodine) from 94 to 40 percent at an estimated cost of $0.10 per person per year. The beauty of this approach to fortification is that it requires no regulatory apparatus for setup or enforcement. It does, however, require annual water pump maintenance.

water iodization altogether at this point. To be able to adapt technology as it goes, a program requires good monitoring, high technical capacity among its staff, and the use of up-to-date information and technology.

Human resource development is intimately related to sustainability. If health workers are sensitized to the effects of micronutrient deficiencies, then prevention will be on a priority list in spite of economic conditions. Institutions and individuals within those institutions need the skills, organizational structures, resources, and reward structures to provide high-quality services. Therefore building institutional capacity—which often requires a long-term commitment—is critical to sustainability.

Habit Formation and Consumer Demand

One underappreciated aspect of sustainability is that once a behavior becomes a habit it is more sustainable. These behaviors include industrial practices, medical routines, provider-client communications, and dietary habits. Integrated programs that generate good medical practices regarding micronutrients are more efficient than vertical programs, which require a single action isolated from specialized workers. Tanzania purposely chose to integrate supplementation into the primary health system because it was concerned about sustainability; as a result, the impact was perhaps less rapid and dramatic, but is likely to last longer than a campaign-type program.

Any behavior needs reinforcement to be perpetuated, but social reinforcement ultimately can replace public health messages. Making conscious the subliminal desires for the benefits of micronutrients and directing demand to appropriate supplements, fortified foods, and natural foods are essential in all micronutrient programs. That demand, in turn, should generate sustainability. If the target beneficiaries think they are entitled to a supplement or a fortified or natural food, then their demands are likely to create political currency and sustain the program.

CHAPTER SEVEN

Success within This Decade

IN September 1990 the World Summit for Children endorsed some challenging goals for micronutrients for the year 2000: virtual elimination of vitamin A and iodine deficiencies and a reduction by one-third of iron deficiency anemia in women.[17] Achieving these goals will require the combined efforts of governments, international organizations, NGOs, and private industry. Consumer education, improvement of supplement delivery infrastructure, and strengthening regulatory systems are the key activities in overcoming micronutrient malnutrition. Complementing these three approaches are programs to increase the supply of micronutrient-rich unprocessed foods. Therefore, work over the remainder of this decade should focus on the following key issues:

1. Raising awareness of leaders of the need to take action against micronutrient malnutrition for economic, political, and humanitarian reasons.

2. Raising consumer demand for micronutrients from pharmaceutical supplements, fortified food, and unprocessed micronutrient-rich food, using policy advocacy, social marketing, and commercial advertising.

3. Improving the effectiveness and coverage of pharmaceutical delivery systems using new outreach mechanisms, better logistics, and improved client counseling.

4. Maximizing industry compliance with fortification mandates through incentives to private industry and through building objective, competent, and respected regulatory enforcement institutions.

5. Designing and managing sustainable programs that are decentralized, enhance institutional capacity and human resources, and monitor performance through management information.

Programs should consider both pharmaceutical supplements and food as sources of micronutrients, but all programs should include nutrition social marketing techniques. Table 7.1 shows a decision matrix for undertaking different kinds of micronutrient programs.

Table 7.1   Decision Matrix and Program Options for Iron, Iodine, and Vitamin A Deficiencies

Deficiencies	Supplementation	Fortification	Dietary Change
Vitamin A	Likely to be needed in short term where prevalence is high. Medical targeting and delivery through EPI desirable.	Not likely to be needed except for refugees, or except where climate and/or dietary traditions exclude major vitamin A food sources from the diet. May be desirable where the ideal food vehicle exists.	Likely to be needed in most deficient countries. Start simultaneously with supplementation. Support, if necessary, with agricultural extension and inputs.
Iodine	Likely to be needed in the short term wherever cretinism exists. In the long term, it may be required in isolated geographical areas where the salt industry is traditional and commercial markets are poorly developed.	Likely to be needed in all deficient countries. May not be immediate solution where the salt industry is dispersed and artisanal.	Unlikely to be of use except over the very long term (until the diet derives from distant, iodine-replete soils, and from certain seafoods).
Iron	Likely to be needed in the short and long term for pregnant women and possibly young children.	Likely to be needed in most countries. Research and development probably needed. Weaning foods need iron fortification.	Most promising where meat is consumed widely and where iron cooking pots used. Agricultural extension to promote livestock production, legumes, and vitamin C foods needed.

Raising Awareness

Despite three major international policy meetings at which micronutrients were high on the agenda, policymakers in many countries still need to be convinced of the imperative to attack micronutrient malnutrition.

Moving leaders to action requires their learning and understanding the costs of micronutrient malnutrition and the cost-benefit ratio of interventions. Many of the lessons described in this book can be used to reassure policymakers that interventions are feasible, affordable, and effective. UNICEF has financed the production of several effective videos on micronutrient malnutrition; the U.S. Agency for International Development (USAID) has developed a computer model to show graphically what micronutrient malnutrition means to a country; and various drug manufacturers and NGOs have developed persuasive print materials and presentations on micronutrients.

These materials, along with personal appeals from agency representatives and advocates, must be shown and given to top political leaders, professional organizations, NGOs, and grass roots organizations. Moreover, the message that micronutrient malnutrition is a serious health problem that can be addressed by specific behaviors must be reinforced in the population at large by health workers, educators, and agricultural extensionists.

Understanding the potential gains from action and experiencing the demand from the public is enough to galvanize the political establishment to action in some countries. The feedback of results to the public and the leadership validates and sustains the resulting programs.

Institutional Development

The ideal delivery infrastructure for pharmaceutical supplements is the public health system, but the health systems in many countries—perhaps most—do not have good coverage of geographic regions and socioeconomic groups at greatest risk (including women). In that event, the health system must be strengthened while other avenues for education and distribution are brought into play alongside it. Other delivery vehicles could be vertical EPI programs, childcare programs, schools, agricultural extensionists, social welfare workers, religious organizations, political organizations, and the commercial pharmaceuticals markets. Public mobilization and education is needed for all of the mechanisms to be effective and efficient.

Fortification for public health purposes should be mandatory and territory-wide, and accompanied by a regulatory apparatus capable of detecting and enforcing compliance with regulations. Technical training and support are important to the functioning of a regulatory system, but more important than anything else is professional integrity. Integrity is essentially a matter of individual values, but, to cultivate and protect those values, a regulatory institution must engender pride and professionalism in its staff. Adequate pay, respect, personal security, and rewards for exemplary performance can reinforce the professional integrity and esprit de corps of regulatory institutions. "Whistle blowing" (reporting misdeeds of colleagues) is an important check on dishonesty. If neither the food industry nor the consumer believes in the regulatory system, it is useless.

It is not necessary to build a complete food control authority in order to monitor compliance with fortification. Where some appropriate administrative unit already exists (generally in the ministry of health or industry or in the bureau of standards), specialized tasks and equipment can be given to it. Otherwise, a new mechanism, such as an independent private laboratory, can be charged with certifying compliance.

In the past, many donor micronutrient programs have been directed from outside the target country and focused on supply, generally of pharmaceutical supplements. Donors must now concentrate on raising political commitment and finding locally appropriate solutions to micronutrient malnutrition.

Each developing country has prepared a national nutrition assessment for the International Conference on Nutrition, and many are preparing action plans. The first priority for donors is to support the further refinement of these national strategies and to support local feasibility studies, training, and technical assistance to help turn those concepts into national programs.

Second, new resources have to be mobilized from governments and donors. At present donors spend barely $50 million per year worldwide on micronutrients (primarily UNICEF and USAID donations of vitamin A and iodine capsules). The worldwide goal for micronutrient sufficiency will never be achieved at that level of spending. The recurrent costs alone to address all deficiencies in the most cost-effective fashion in all deficient countries are estimated to be $1 billion per year. Clearly, consumers will pay some of these costs, but the residual costs plus start-up costs far exceed the current government and donor expenditures. New donors, as well as NGOs and industry, must be mobilized and greater weight placed on feasibility studies, training, monitoring, and micronutrient social marketing.

The World Bank's Role

Until recently, the World Bank has not been a major donor in micronutrients. Recent investments in salt iodization, basic health packages that include micronutrient supplements, and nutritional social marketing, however, have established a niche for the Bank, particularly in attracting political support, effecting

Table 7.2 Incorporating Micronutrients into Selected World Bank Operations

| | Sector analysis | | | |
	Factors that affect MN malnutrition	Factors affected by MN malnutrition	Policy levers	Investment opportunities
Poverty and food security	Analyze how lack of purchasing power limits access to a varied diet.	Estimate handicaps and lost work productivity due to MN deficiencies.	Improve qualitative consumption effects of wage and employment policies, tax and welfare policies, and consumer food price policies; micro-credit access.	Introduce or improve safety nets for the poor that address qualitative as well as quantitative nutritional needs; microcredit schemes plus consumer education.
Health sector	Estimate the contributions of parasites, high fertility, inadequate breast feeding, diarrhea, and measles to deficiencies in some or all MN deficiencies.	Estimate excess morbidity and mortality due to vitamin A deficiency and blindness, anemia, and IDD.	Improve health policy so it includes norms, training, monitoring, and treatment of nutrient deficiencies; rational drug use to include MN supplements; and drug supply management reforms to include MN supplements.	Improve health system delivery of supplements; enforce fortification; monitor MN status; finance nutrition education and deworming.
Education sector		Examine educational inefficiencies caused by anemia, vitamin A blindness, and IDD-induced mental retardation and deaf-mutism.	Broaden criteria for school-readiness of students to include nutritional status; train teachers about MN malnutrition; allocate adequate resources to school nutrition.	Include modules in education projects to treat school children (deworming, MN supplements, school feeding); make capital investments in school kitchens; TA and extension for school gardens.

Food and agriculture sector	Examine production, marketing, and trade policies for effects on quality (nutrients) as well as quantity (calories) of food consumed.	Estimate adverse effects of MN deficiency on agricultural productivity.	Anticipate consequences of food, trade, and financial policies on MN and, if necessary, reform to improve impact.	Invest in consumer education; technical assistance; capital investments; agricultural research and extension focused on MN.
Industry	Determine the effects of the food industry on nutritional quality of diet. Analyze the incentives and disincentives for producing nutritious food (including fortified food).	Estimate lost productivity due to anemia and IDD; estimate workforce disabled by MN deficiencies.	Develop and enforce regulations that promote nutrition and provide level playing field (content, labeling); certification of quality. Remove trade barriers and regulatory barriers to food industry development.	Support public marketing campaigns for "good" foods; public capital investment and equipment (especially for quality control and fortification).
Infrastructure (water, roads)	Assess whether water can be used to deliver MN at household, village, or municipal level; market access.	Determine role of contaminated water in MN depletion.	Facilitate fortification of well water or public water supplies.	Make capital investments in water fortification; food market infrastructure.

MN   Micronutrient.
IDD Iodine deficiency disorders.
TA   Technical assistance.

cross-sectoral policy reforms, and building bridges between public and private sectors to bring about fortification. Taking advantage of this momentum, future solutions to micronutrient malnutrition should be considered an integral part of the World Bank country assistance strategy, including sector work, policy dialogue, and the investment program (illustrated in Table 7.2). Even in non-social sectors—like industry and infrastructure—highly cost-effective interventions have been implemented on a large scale. Every appropriate World Bank project should include a micronutrient intervention where micronutrient malnutrition exists (Appendix Table A.3) and the project provides a framework for it when the problem is not being addressed adequately by other actions. The Bank complements quite well the other major donors in this area. Using its financial resources as well as its traditional strengths of economic analysis and management, the Bank can play a key role in supporting the appropriate roles for private food industry, public institutions, and the consumers. Because it is not a technical institution, the Bank coordinates closely with other donors, private industry, the academic community, and local experts to assure high-quality design and implementation. The Bank was a founding member of the Micronutrient Initiative, a multidonor mechanism to support feasibility studies, country assessments, and global communications to accelerate the resolution of micronutrient malnutrition.

Biochemical and Social Research

Aside from general feasibility studies to adapt technology to the specific needs of a country and the social marketing research that must inform a sustainable micronutrient program, more basic research is needed on certain key issues.

The medical community needs a better understanding of dosages and nutrient/immunization interactions in children under 6 months of age. In addition, research and development work should focus on diagnostic tools for vitamin A deficiency that are rapid, acceptable to the client, and appropriate to field conditions; cheap, simple, semiquantitative assessment techniques for verification of iron and vitamin A levels in fortified foods; and long-lasting iron supplements with no side effects.

Operations research, preferable on actual programs, could yield better information on the costs, cost-effectiveness, and social and economic benefits of micronutrient interventions, particularly of nutrition education.

Summary

Vitamin and mineral deficiencies deprive 1 billion people worldwide of their intellect, strength, and vitality. For less than 0.3 percent of their GDP, nutrient-deficient countries could rid themselves of these entirely preventable diseases, which now cost them more than 5 percent of their GDP in lost lives, disability, and productivity. No country with micronutrient malnutrition can afford *not* to take action. This book has reviewed the lessons of experience in implementing micronutrient programs. If political will, adequate technical and financial support, and these lessons are applied, micronutrient malnutrition can be reduced significantly throughout the world within this generation.

Notes

1. Some other nutrients, including zinc, certain B vitamins, and calcium, are probably deficient in many developing countries, but the tools for detecting the problem are inadequate.

2. Rising income first allows greater consumption of staple grains and legumes, which contain low-quality (not readily absorbed) iron. A further rise in income permits the substitution of meat (where religion does not forbid it), which has higher-quality iron, and hence the absorption of iron in the diet increases. Even if intake from grain sources decreases among the wealthy, the meat raises the intake of net usable iron (Behrman and Deolalikar 1987; Bouis 1992; Kennedy and Payongayong 1991; Meesook and Chernichovsky 1984).

3. Other interventions with costs ranging between these two include case management of acute respiratory infection, diarrheal control via breastfeeding promotion and improved weaning, polio immunization, helminth (hookworm) control, immunizations for measles, and fertility control.

4. Even if some supplies are available locally, international competitive procurement yields the best price and quality. UNICEF, for example, buys potassium iodate (for salt iodation) for less than $10 per kilogram compared with prices of $20 to $30 per kilogram.

5. The SCN is the Sub-Committee on Nutrition of the UN Administrative Coordinating Committee, which convened a meeting on iron deficiency in Dublin during June 1990.

6. Excessive intakes of vitamin A, iodine, and iron can have severe side effects but rarely have these been frequent enough to cause concern. A surprising fact is that the megadose capsules are not the most toxic but rather the iron tablets, which can be deadly when consumed in large quantities by young children.

7. In Bangladesh, the Small and Cottage Industries Corporation, which licenses and regulates salt producers and refiners, is charged with the responsibility for implementing the iodization program and monitoring it at the production level. Retail and

consumer level monitoring will have to be the responsibility of the ministry of health through the provincial or district health network.

8. This strategy has been effective in Bolivia through a state-run salt marketing company (Emcosal). Voluntary regulation was not effective in Kenya, however, where legal loopholes left almost half of the salt unfortified. Only after enactment of mandatory fortification was a credible portion of the salt iodized.

9. One might argue in favor of consumer choice as an absolute right, but that argument would seem to oppose health and safety regulations of all sorts. In this case, society as a whole benefits from fortification, the benefits exceed the costs manyfold, and directing consumer choice to the socially preferred good (the fortified product) would be more expensive and take far longer than limiting consumer choice. Finally, consumer (citizen) support is ultimately necessary if the fortification program as a whole (including enforcement) is to work and if the larger micronutrient program, of which it is a part, is to work.

10. Algeria had hoped for years that regional iodization of salt would suffice. But because the regions not covered probably also had low iodine levels, universal fortification would have been more practical and economical than the regional approach. In 1991 Algeria acknowledged its failure, and the legislature passed a law requiring nationwide iodization. Now Algeria is considered to be a model for salt iodization.

11. Food sources of vitamin C (which enhances iron absorption) and A and, to some extent, iron, are inexpensive, culturally acceptable, and widely available. The trouble is that they are not given to the most vulnerable individuals, household storage is difficult, or they are unavailable seasonally. The most important dietary sources of these nutrients are dark green leafy vegetables, yellow and orange fruits and vegetables, legumes, and red meat. Some of these foods are cultivated and others are foraged. Among the cultivated foods are tree crops (fruits, red oil palm, and edible leaf trees), legumes, field crops (horticultural crops, leaves of tubers, and yellow-fleshed tubers), and small livestock. The foraged foods such as wild fruits and berries, small animals, and green leaves, tend to be trapped or picked in uncultivated land and forests.

12. Haiti and Senegal have developed dried mango as a local industry for women and as an economical way to preserve a highly seasonal food that is rich in vitamin A.

13. When women in Nepal were encouraged to manage their own forests, they were able to protect wild foods they depended on (FAO 1990).

14. The fortification of MSG with vitamin A was launched with the hope that it would be a significant program, but technical difficulties and political resistance have prevented national implementation. The key strategy of the government regarding iodine has been to iodize all salt, but compliance is still low; recent indications are that salt iodization will soon be a major effort. Iodized oil injections, seen as a short-term cross-sectoral program for high-risk areas, have had high but decreasing coverage since they were initiated in 1974. The government has dealt with iron deficiency least effectively, and the government strategy relies virtually exclusively on getting pregnant women to take iron pills.

15. Taking blood, for instance, should be avoided if possible. If blood is taken at all, it should be analyzed for all three micronutrient deficiencies at once. If successful, a

new technology for assessing the three deficiencies from spots of blood on filter paper will be a major breakthrough.

16. One creative monitoring system was used in Guatemala for sugar fortification with vitamin A. Because vitamin A status is best measured by liver stores of the nutrient, human liver samples were taken from a cross-section of cadavers in the country and showed quite well the coverage of the fortification program. The process was less expensive than a survey but required access to a truly representative sample of cadavers.

17. These goals were subsequently reaffirmed at the "Ending Hidden Hunger" policy conference in October 1991 and at the International Conference on Nutrition in December 1992.

Appendix A. Prevalence Data

Table A.1 Micronutrient Malnutrition as a Public Health Problem
(number of countries, latest data)

Countries with	Vitamin A and iron deficiencies	Iodine and iron deficiencies	Vitamin A and iodine and iron deficiencies	Iron deficiencies	No micro-nutrient deficiencies
More than 20 percent undernutrition	9	8	22	9	1
Less than 20 percent undernutrition	2	13	2	28	3
No data on under-nutrition	0	6	5	8	4

Source: ICCIDD 1990; WHO 1988; ACC/SCN 1992. See Table A.3.

Table A.2 Status of Country Programs
(number of comprehensive national micronutrient programs and number of countries with problems)

Region	Iodine	Vitamin A	Iron
Africa	0/41	0/43	0/45
Americas	8/19	4/17	6/32
Southeast Asia	0/10	0/8	0/11
Europe	10/30	—	—
Eastern Mediterranean	0/10	—	—
West Pacific	3/21	0/9	5/23

— Not available.
Source: WHO 1992, Table 2.

Table A.3   Developing Countries with Micronutrient Deficiency Disorders

	Micronutrient deficiencies			
Area	*Vitamin A*[a] *and iron*[b]	*Iodine*[c] *and iron*	*Vitamin A, iron, and iodine*	*Iron only*[d]
Africa				
Countries with > 20 percent children underweight[e]	Burundi Mauritania Niger Rwanda Uganda	CAR Comoros Congo Madagascar Senegal Sierra Leone	Benin Burkina Faso Ethiopia Ghana Kenya Malawi Mali Mozambique Nigeria Sudan Tanzania Zambia	Guinea-Bissau Liberia Mauritius Somalia (S. Africa) Togo
Countries with < 20 percent children underweight[e]		Botswana Cameroon Côte d'Ivoire Lesotho Zaire Zimbabwe		Cape Verde Gabon Gambia São Tomé/ Principe Seychelles Swaziland
Countries with unknown percent of children underweight[e]		Guinea Namibia	Angola Chad	Djibouti Eq. Guinea
Asia				
Countries with > 20 percent children underweight[e]	PNG Thailand	Malaysia	Bangladesh India Indonesia Lao P.D.R. Myanmar Nepal Sri Lanka Viet Nam	Maldives

Table A.3 (*continued*)

Area	Micronutrient deficiencies			
	Vitamin A[a] *and iron*[b]	*Iodine*[c] *and iron*	*Vitamin A, iron, and iodine*	*Iron only*[d]
Asia (continued)				
Countries with < 20 percent children underweight[e]	Kiribati		Philippines	Fiji F. Polynesia (Korea, Republic) Singapore Solomon Isl. Vanuatu W. Samoa
Countries with unknown percent of children underweight[e]		China	Bhutan Kampuchea	(Korea D.) Mongolia
Middle East				
Countries with > 20 percent children underweight[e]		Iran	Pakistan	Yemen
Countries with < 20 percent children underweight[e]		Tunisia		Egypt Jordan Kuwait Lebanon Libya (Palest. Ref.)
Countries with unknown percent of children underweight[e]		Algeria Iraq	Afghanistan	Oman (Qatar) (S. Arabia) Syria Turkey (U.A.E.)

(*Table continues on the following page.*)

Table A.3 (*continued*)

| Area | Micronutrient deficiencies | | | |
	Vitamin A[a] and iron[b]	Iodine[c] and iron	Vitamin A, iron, and iodine	Iron only[d]
Latin America				
Countries with > 20 percent children underweight[e]	Haiti Honduras		Guatemala	Guyana
Countries with < 20 percent children underweight[e]	Brazil	Bolivia Ecuador Mexico Paraguay Peru	Salvador	Antigua Barbados (Chile) Colombia Costa Rica Dominica Dom. Rep. Panama St. Lucia St. Vincent Trinidad/ Tobago (Uruguay)
Countries with unknown percent of children underweight[e]		Venezuela		Argentina Cuba

a. WHO 1988.
b. All developing countries.
c. ICCIDD 1990; Hetzel 1988.
d. In countries with parentheses there is some evidence that iron deficiency is not a public health problem.
e. Galloway 1991. Underweight is defined as less than 2 standard deviations below the mean of the reference standard weight-for-age.

Appendix B.   Methods and Assumptions for Cost-Effectiveness Calculations

This Appendix is excerpted from Levin, Pollitt, Galloway, and McGuire 1993; the tables have been renumbered.

Criteria of Effectiveness

Some interventions will have a high success rate in obtaining repletion, such as injected or oral iodinated oil or oral capsules of vitamin A. Once ingested or injected, these interventions are almost invariably associated with iodine or vitamin A repletion. In contrast, medicinal supplementation with iron or dietary fortification does not always ensure repletion. Because the capacity of the body to store iron is limited, iron supplementation requires that the participant take iron daily. When administered in schools or workplaces, this compliance can be readily maintained. When it is necessary to depend on households continually to take iron supplements, it is not realistic to expect a high level of compliance. Thus the cost of delivering the iron to households is not equivalent to the cost of obtaining iron repletion. Indeed, obtaining compliance may require continuing reinforcement through monitoring and persuasion by village health teams and other educational efforts.

The same is true with fortification. Not only is it necessary for all persons at risk to consume adequate amounts of the fortified food, but the food must have sufficient amounts of the micronutrient at the time of consumption. There may be a compliance problem when unfortified, local products compete with the nationally or regionally distributed fortified ones. In Ecuador it was necessary to mount a social marketing campaign to increase use of a fortified product such as iodinated salt because alternative salt sources were available at the local level (Manoff 1987). In tropical areas the hygroscopic nature of salt that is used for iodine fortification means that unless contained in watertight packaging until consumption, at least some of the iodine will be lost. Iodinated salt in jute bags showed a loss of three-quarters of its iodine in nine months ([Venkatesh] Mannar 1987). The type of packaging, the time it takes to get to consumers, and the use of open or closed containers by shops and consumers will determine potency. In very humid climates with highly undependable transportation and long periods before sale or consumption in open containers, the salt may lose virtually all its iodine. . . .

Cost-Benefit Analysis

. . . . Although it would be desirable to have a standard cost-benefit methodology with precise rules for calculation for every situation, this is not the present case. . . . [A]lthough the conceptual methods for identifying and measuring benefits are well established (Creese and Henderson 1980; Mills 1985), the application of these methods depends crucially on a variety of judgments on both the measurement of benefits and their values. Some of the best work on cost-benefit analysis in the health sector is found in the area of immunization (Creese and Henderson 1980; Creese 1983), and many of the methods used there can be applied to micronutrients.

The basic method of estimating benefits is to identify the positive effects of micronutrient interventions on such areas as morbidity, work output, and educational benefits for children. The benefits of reduced morbidity are generally considered to be the savings in health care and the value of lost productivity; the benefits of work output can be measured with respect to additional days of productive work (in the labor market or household) and the additional productivity per day; and educational benefits include the value of additional student achievement and the reduction in the cost of special educational services or grade repetition. Some of these benefits also have implications for costs. For example, if iron-replete workers are able to put out more work effort to increase productivity, they will also need additional food to compensate for the higher expenditure of energy (Levin 1985, 1986).

. . .[E]ach of the micronutrient interventions has an effect on health, productivity, and other aspects of behavior. In theory, it is only necessary to translate the effects into benefits and to place monetary values on them to compare them with the costs of an intervention. Unfortunately, the lack of field trials that incorporate data collection in the various benefit domains limits the application of cost-benefit analysis to this area. Nevertheless, there exist studies for each of the three micronutrients that are both informative and suggest high returns. . . .

Costs and Benefits

The tables in this appendix show the costs and benefits of various interventions.

Table B.1 Assumptions in Calculating Costs per Disability-Adjusted Life-Year, Death Averted and Income Enhancement

Parameter	Value
Program effectiveness (percent)	75[a]
Unemployment (percent)	25[b]
Life expectancy (years)	70
Discount rate (percent)	3
Annual wage rate (U.S. dollars)	500
Population (number)	100,000
Age distribution (number)	
0–1 year	3,900
1–2 years	3,250
2–3 years	2,340
3–4 years	1,950
4–5 years	1,560
5–9 years	12,000
10–14 years	9,000
15–59 years	57,000[c]
60 years and older	7,000
Malnutrition rates (number and percent)	
PEM	
Children younger than 5	3,900 (30)
Adults stunted from childhood malnutrition	17,000 (30)
Iron	
Anemic children under 15	18,000 (50)
Anemic adult men	7,250 (25)
Anemic pregnant women	2,520 (63)
Total population anemic	49,000
Iodine	
Population deficient	24,000 (24)
Cretinism	50 (0.4)[d]
Vitamin A	
Deficient children under 6	1,950 (15)
Severely deficient children under 6	40 (.27)
Severely deficient children under 6 dying	20 (.16)
Partially blind children under 6	81 (0.060)
Totally blind children under 6	41 (0.028)

(Table continues on the following page.)

Table B.1 (*continued*)

Parameter	Value
Annual deaths from malnutrition (number)	
PEM-related causes in children under 5	160
Severe anemia in women at childbirth	10
Stillbirths related to iodine deficiency	10
Neonatal deaths related to iodine deficiency	10
Children under 5 with vitamin A deficiency	40
Degree of disability (percent)[e]	
Undernutrition	10
Iron deficiency	20
Iodine deficiency	5
Cretinism	50
Partial blindness	25
Total blindness	50

a. Includes coverage as well as efficacy.
b. Adults ages 15–59.
c. Includes 25,000 women of reproductive age, of whom 4,000 are pregnant.
d. One child is born with cretinism each year.
e. Health and productivity disability.
Source: Based on author's assumptions.

Table B.2   Nutrition Program Costs for Population of 10,000

Intervention	Target group	Annual per capita cost (US$)	Annual program cost (US$)
Food supplements	Pregnant women Children 0–3 years	46.0	620,540
Nutrition education	Pregnant women	2.0	26,980
Food subsidy	Bottom quintile	30.0	600,000
Integrated nutrition PHC	Pregnant women	25.0	337,250
School feeding	Children 5–9 years	12.0	144,000
Iron			
Supplement[a]	Pregnant women	2.0	8,000
Fortification	Entire population	0.2	20,000
Iodine			
Supplement, selective	Women	0.5	12,500
Supplement, total	Entire	0.5	23,250
Fortification	Entire population	0.1	10,000
Vitamin A			
Supplement	Children 0–5 years	0.5	6,500
Fortification	Entire population	0.2	20,000

Note: Based on assumptions in Table B.1.
a. Assumes six prenatal visits plus 200 iron tablets.
Source: Ho 1985; Levin 1985; Kennedy and Alderman 1987.

Table B.3   Assumptions in Calculating Costs and Effectiveness
of Iron Interventions

Parameter	Iron supplementation of pregnant women	Iron fortification
Target group	Pregnant women	All people
Number	4,000	100,000
Average rate (percent)[a]	63	50
Per capita cost (US$)[b]	2	0.20
Program effectiveness (percent)	75	75
Deaths averted	10	10
Immediate productivity gains (percent)	20	20
Program duration (days)	200	Year round
Program costs (US$)	8,000	20,000
Discounted wage gains (US$)	221,280[c]	1,682,720[d]
DALY gained	624[e]	4,520[f]
Wage gains divided by program cost	27.7	84.1
Cost per DALY (US$)	12.8	4.40
Cost per death averted (US$)	800	2,000

Note: Based on assumptions in Table B.1.
a. Rate of anemia for iron supplementation of pregnant women; rate of iron deficiency for iron fortification.
b. Per pregnancy for iron supplementation; per participant for iron fortification.
c. Calculated as the product of the number of anemic participants times disability times wages times effectiveness times employment, plus the product of number of deaths times wage times employment times productive life expectancy: ([0.63 x 3,990] x 0.2 x 500 x 0.75 x 0.75) + (10 x 500 x 0.75 x 21.3) = 141,400 + 79,880 = 221,280.
d. Calculated as the product of the number of adult participants times the rate of anemia times disability times effectiveness times employment times wage, plus the product of the number of deaths times wage times employment times productive life expectancy: (56,990 x 0.5 x 0.2 x 0.75 x 500) + (10 x 500 x 0.75 x 21.3) = 1,602,840 + 79,880 = 1,682,720.
e. Calculated as the product of the number of deaths times life expectancy, plus the product of disability times number of malnourished participants times effectiveness: (10 x 24.7) + (0.2 x 0.63 x 3,990 x 0.75) = 247 + 377 = 624.
f. Calculated as the product of number of adult participants times the rate of anemia times disability times effectiveness, plus the product of the number of deaths times life expectancy: (56,990 x 0.5 x 0.2 x 0.75) + (10 x 24.7) = 4,270 + 250 = 4,520.
Source: Based on author's assumptions.

Table B.4   Costs and Effectiveness of Iodine Interventions

Parameter	Iodine supplement: targeted coverage	Iodine supplement: mass coverage	Iodization of salt or water
Target group	Reproductive-age women	Everyone under age 60	Everyone
Number	25,000	93,000	100,000
Average rate of iodine deficiency (percent)	24	24	24
Per capita cost (US$)[a]	0.50	0.50	0.10
Program effectiveness (percent)	75[b]	75	75
Deaths averted	10[c]	10	10
Productivity loss (percent)			
Normal population	5	5	5
Cretins	50	50	50
Program duration	Year round	Year round	Year round
Program costs (US$)	12,500	46,500	100,000
Discounted wage gains (US$)	172,000[d]	280,000[e]	280,000[e]
DALY gained	660[f]	1,270[g]	1,335[h]
Wage gains divided by program cost (US$)	13.8	6.0	28
Cost per DALY (US$)	18.9	37	7.5
Cost per death averted (US$)	1,250	4,650	1,000

Note: Based on assumptions in Table B.1.
a. Per participant per year.
b. Prevents both neonatal death and cretinism.
c. Neonatal.
d. Calculated as the product of the number of participants times the rate of deficiency times disability times wage times effectiveness times employment rate, plus number who died times productive life expectancy times employment rate times wage for ten cretins, plus the product of frequency times productive life expectancy times employment times wages for ten deaths: (25,000 x 0.24 x 0.05 x 500 x 0.75 x 0.75) + (10 x 0.5 x 15.5765 x 0.75 x 500) + (10 x 15.5765 x 0.75 x 500) = 84,380 + 29,210 + 58,410 = 172,000.
e. Calculated as in note d: (57,000 x 0.24 x 0.05 x 500 x 0.75 x 0.75) + (10 x 0.5 x 15.5765 x 0.75 x 500) + (10 x 15.5765 x 0.75 x 500) = 192,380 + 29,210 + 58,410 = 280,000.
f. Calculated as the product of the number of participants times the rate of deficiency times disability times effectiveness, plus the product of disability times life expectancy for ten cretins, plus the life expectancy for ten deaths: (25,000 x 0.24 x 0.05 x 0.75) + (10 x 0.5 x 29) + 10 x 29 = 225 + 145 + 290 = 660.
g. Calculated as in note f: (93,000 x 0.24 x 0.05 x 0.75) + (10 x 0.5 x 29) + 10 x 29 = 837 + 145 + 290 = 1,270.
h. Calculated as in note f: (99,980 x 0.24 x 0.05 x 0.75) + (10 x 0.5 x 29) + 10 x 29 = 900 + 145 + 290 = 1,335.
Source: Based on author's assumptions.

Table B.5   Costs and Effectiveness of Vitamin A Intervention

Parameter	Vitamin A supplementation[a]	Vitamin A fortification
Target group	Children under 5	Entire population
Number	13,000	100,000
Average rate of vitamin A deficiency (percent)[b]	15	15
Per capita cost (US$)[c]	0.50	0.20
Program effectiveness (percent)	75	75
Deaths averted (number)	20	20
Blindness averted (number)		
Total	4	4
Partial	8	8
Productivity loss (percent)		
Totally blind	50	50
Partially blind	25	25
Program duration	Year round	Year round
Program costs (US$)	6,500	20,000
Discounted wage gains (US$)	140,188[d]	140,188[d]
DALY gained	696[e]	696[e]
Wage gain divided by program cost	21.6	7.0
Cost per DALY (US$)	9.3	29
Cost per death averted (US$)	325	1,000

Note: Based on assumptions in Table B.1.
a. Semiannual mass dose.
b. In children under 5 years.
c. Per participant.
d. Does not include losses due to excess child morbidity. Calculated as the product of the number of deaths averted times the productive life expectancy times employment times wage, plus the product of the number of total blindness averted times productive life expectancy times disability times employment times wage, plus the product of the number of partial blindness averted times productive life expectancy times disability times employment times wage: (20 x 15.5765 x 0.75 x 500) + (4 x 15.5765 x 0.5 x 0.75 x 500) + (8 x 15.5765 x 0.25 x 0.75 x 500) = 116,824 + 11,682 + 11,682 = 140,188.
e. Calculated as deaths averted times discounted remaining life expectancy plus total blindness times disability times discounted remaining life expectancy plus partial blindness times disability times discounted remaining life expectancy: (20 x 29) + (4 x 0.5 x 29) + (8 x 0.25 x 29) = 696.
Source: Based on author's assumptions.

Bibliography

The word "processed" describes informally reproduced works that may not be commonly available through libraries.

ACC/SCN (Administrative Committee on Coordination/SubCommittee on Nutrition). 1989. "Nutrition in Times of Disaster." *SCN News* 3: 11–13 (Geneva).

_____. 1991. "Controlling Iron Deficiency." ACC/SCN State-of-the-Art Series, Nutrition Policy Discussion Paper 9. United Nations ACC/SCN, Geneva.

_____. 1992. *Second Report on the World Nutrition Situation*. Vol. I, "Global and Regional Results." Prepared in collaboration with the International Food Policy Research Institute. Washington, D.C.

Acharya, S. 1991. "Supplementation of Iodine and Vitamin A with Reference to Nepal." *Ending Hidden Hunger Meeting Proceedings*. Task Force on Child Survival, Montreal, Canada, October 10–12.

Bates, C. J., H. J. Powers, W. H. Lamb, W. Gelman, and E. Webb. 1987. "Effect of Supplementary Vitamins and Iron on Malaria Indices in Rural Gambian Children." *Transcripts of Royal Society of Tropical Medicine and Hygiene* 81: 286–91.

Beaton, G. H., R. Martorell, K. A. L'Abbe, B. Edmonston, G. McCabe, A. C. Ross, and B. Harvey. 1993. "Effectiveness of Vitamin A Supplementation in the Control of Young Child Morbidity and Mortality in Developing Countries. Summary Report." A project of the International Nutrition Program, Department of Nutritional Sciences, Faculty of Medicine, University of Toronto, Toronto, Canada.

Behrman, J. R., and A. B. Deolalikar. 1987. "Will Developing Country Nutrition Improve with Income? A Case Study for Rural South India." *Journal of Political Economy* 95(3): 492–507.

Bouis, H. W. 1992. "The Determinants of Household-Level Demand for Micronutrients: An Analysis for Philippine Farm Households." Report written for the World Bank, Population and Human Resources Department, Population, Health, and Nutrition Division. Processed. Washington, D.C.

Bundy, D. A. P., and J. M. Del Rosso. 1993. "Making Nutrition Improvements at Low Cost Through Parasite Control." HRO Working Paper 7. World Bank, Human Resources Development and Operations Policy Vice-Presidency, Washington, D.C.

Burnham, G. 1992. "Treatment of Malaria in Pregnancy." *PVO Child Survival Technical Report* 3(1): 9–11.

Byles, A., and A. D'Sa. 1970. "Reduction of the Reaction Due to Iron Dextran Infusion Using Chloroquine." *British Medical Journal* 3: 625–27.

CDC (Centers for Disease Control). 1992. *Famine-Affected, Refugee, and Displaced Populations: Recommendations for Public Health Issues.* Morbidity and Mortality Weekly Report 41: RR-13. Washington, D.C.: U.S. Department of Health and Human Services, Public Health Service.

Chippaux, J-P., D. Schneider, A. Aplogan, J-L. Dyck, J. Berger. 1991. "Iron Supplementation Effect on Malaria Infection."*Bulletin de la Société de Pathologie Exotique* 84(1): 54–62.

Clugston, G., E. Dulberg, C. Pandav, R. Tilden. 1987. "Iodine Deficiency Disorders in South East Asia." In B. Hetzel, J. Dunn, and J. Stanbury, eds., *The Prevention and Control of Iodine Deficiency Disorders.* Amsterdam: Elsevier.

Cohen, N., H. Rahman, J. Sprague, M. A. Jalil, E. Leemhuis de Regt, and M. Mitra. 1985. "Prevalence and Determinants of Nutritional Blindness in Bangladeshi Children." *World Health Statistics Quarterly* 38: 317–30.

Creese, A. L. 1983. "The Economic Evaluation of Immunization Programmes." In K. Lee and A. Mills, eds., *The Economics of Health in Developing Countries*. New York: Oxford University Press.

_____, and R. H. Henderson. 1980. "Cost-Benefit Analysis and Immunization Programmes in Developing Countries." *Bulletin of WHO* 58: 491-97.

DeMaeyer, E. 1989. *Preventing and Controlling Iron Deficiency Anemia Through Primary Health Care: A Guide for Health Administrators and Programme Managers.* Geneva: World Health Organization.

Eastman, S. 1987. "Vitamin A: Deficiency and Xerophthalmia." *Assignment Children* 3. New York: UNICEF.

FAO (Food and Agriculture Organization of the United Nations). 1990. *Women in Agricultural Development: Women and Food Systems in Agriculture.* Rome: FAO, Women in Agricultural Production and Rural Development Service, Human Resources, Institutions, and Agrarian Reform Division.

Fleming, A. F. 1987. "Maternal Anaemia in Northern Nigeria: Causes and Solutions." *World Health Forum* 8(3): 339–43.

_____. 1989. "The Aetiology of Severe Anaemia in Pregnancy in Ndola, Zambia." *Annals of Tropical Medicine and Parasitology* 83(1): 37–49.

Frankenberger, T., M. Stone, and S. Saenz de Tejada. 1989. "Household Vegetable Gardens in Africa: Case Studies from Mauritania and Lesotho." *Arid Lands Newsletter* 29: 21–24.

Galloway, R. 1991. "Global Indicators of Nutritional Risk." PRE Working Paper 591. World Bank, Population, Health, and Nutrition Department, Washington, D.C.

Gross, R. N., and R. L. Tilden. 1988. "Vitamin A Cost-Effectiveness Model." *International Health Planning and Management* 3: 225–44.

Harvey, P. W. J., P. F. Heywood, M. C. Nesheim, K. Galme, M. Zegans, J-P. Habicht, L. S. Stephenson, K. L. Radimer, B. Brabin, K. Forsyth, and M. P. Alpers. 1989. "The Effect of Iron Therapy on Malarial Infection in Papua New Guinean Schoolchildren." *American Journal of Tropical Medicine* 40(1): 12–18.

Hetzel, B. S. 1988. The Prevention and Control of Iodine Deficiency Disorders. ACC/SCN State-of-the-Art Series. Nutrition Policy Discussion Paper 3. United Nations ACC/SCN, Geneva.

———. 1989. *The Story of Iodine Deficiency*. Delhi: Oxford University Press. pp. 91–99.

Ho, T. J. 1985. "Economic Issues in Assessing Nutrition Projects: Costs, Affordability, and Cost-Effectiveness." PHN Technical Note 85-14. World Bank, Population, Health, and Nutrition Department, Washington, D.C.

Hunt, J. R., L. M. Mullen, G. I. Lykken, S. K. Gallagher, and F. H. Nielsen. 1990. "Ascorbic Acid: Effect on Ongoing Iron Absorption and Status in Iron-Depleted Young Women." *American Journal of Clinical Nutrition* 51: 649–55.

ICCIDD (International Council for the Control of Iodine Deficiency Disorders). 1990. *Global Action Plan for Elimination of IDD as a Major Public Health Problem by the Year 2000*. Processed. Adelaide, Australia: ICCIDD.

Jamison, D. T. 1993. "Disease Control Priorities in Developing Countries: An Overview." In D. T. Jamison, W. H. Mosley, A. R. Measham, and J. L. Bobadilla, eds., *Disease Control Priorities in Developing Countries*. New York: Oxford University Press for the World Bank.

Jelliffe, E. 1992. "Materno-Fetal Malaria: Multiple Dyadic Dilemmas." In E. Wijeyaratne, E. Rathgeber, and E. St.-Onge, eds., *Women and Tropical Diseases*. Ottawa, Canada: International Development Research Centre, UNDP/World Bank/WHO Special Programme for Research and Training in Tropical Diseases.

Kennedy, E., and E. Payongayong. 1991. "Patterns of Macronutrient and Micronutrient Consumption and Implications for Monitoring and Evaluating." Report supported by the Food and Nutrition Monitoring Project funded by the United States Agency for International Development, Office of Nutrition, Washington, D.C.

Kennedy, E. T., and H. H. Alderman. 1987. *Comparative Analyses of Nutritional Effectiveness of Food Subsidies and Other Food-Related Interventions*. Washington, D.C.: International Food Policy Research Institute.

Lakritz, E. M., C. C. Campbell, and T. K. Ruebush II. 1992. "Effect of Blood Transfusion on Survival Among Children in a Kenyan Hospital." *Lancet* 340: 524–28.

Levin, H. M. 1985. *A Benefit-Cost Analysis of Nutritional Interventions for Anemia Reduction*. PHN Technical Note 85-12. World Bank, Population, Health, and Nutrition Department, Washington, D.C.

———. 1986. A Benefit-Cost Analysis of Nutritional Programmes for Anemia Reduction. *World Bank Research Observer* 1(2): 219–45.

Levin, H., E. Pollitt, R. Galloway, and J. McGuire. 1993. "Micronutrient Deficiency Disorders." In D. T. Jamison, W. H. Mosley, A. R. Measham, and J. L. Bobadilla, eds., *Disease Control Priorities in Developing Countries*. New York: Oxford University Press for the World Bank.

Lozoff, B., E. Jimenez, and A. Wolf 1991. "Long-term Developmental Outcomes of Infants With Iron Deficiency." *New England Journal of Medicine* 325: 687–94.

MacFarlane, B. J., W. B. Vander Riet, T. H. Bothwell, R. D. Baynes, D. Sieganberg, U. Schmidt, A. Tal, J. R. Tayler, and F. Mayet. 1990. "Effects of Traditional Oriental Soy Products on Iron Absorption." *American Journal of Clinical Nutrition* 51: 873–80.

Manoff, R. K. 1987. "Social Marketing: New Tool to Combat Iodine Deficiency Disorders." In B. S. Hetzel, J. T. Dunn, and J. B. Stanbury, eds., *The Prevention and Control of Iodine Deficiency Disorders*. New York: Elsevier.

Masawe, A., J. Muindi, and G. Swai. 1974. "Infections in Iron Deficiency and Other Types of Anemia in the Tropics." *Lancet* 2: 314–17.

Meesook, O. A., and D. Chernichovsky. 1984. "Patterns of Food Consumption and Nutrition in Indonesia." Staff Working Paper 670. World Bank, Development Economics Department, Washington, D.C.

Mills, A. 1985. "Economic Evaluation of Health Programmes: Application of the Principles in Developing Countries." *World Health Statistics Quarterly* 38: 368-82.

Neumann, C. 1991. "Analysis of CRSP Data in Kenya for the Population, Health and Nutrition Division." Consultant report using data collected in the Collaborative Research Support Program in Nutrition for USAID. World Bank, Population and Human Resources Department, Population, Health, and Nutrition Division, Washington, D.C.

Oppenheimer, S. 1989. "Iron and Infection: The Clinical Evidence." *Acta Paediatrica Scandinavica* (Suppl.) 361: 53–62.

Oppenheimer, S. J., F. D. Gibson, S. B. MacFarlane, J. B. Moody, C. Harrison, A. Spencer, and O. Bunari. 1986. "Iron Supplementation Increases Prevalence and Effects of Malaria: Report on Clinical Studies in Papua New Guinea." *Transcripts of Royal Society of Tropical Medicine and Hygiene* 80: 603–12.

_____. 1989. "Total Dose Iron Infusion, Malaria, and Pregnancy in Papua New Guinea." *Transcripts of Royal Society of Tropical Medicine and Hygiene* 5: 818–22.

Pollitt, E., P. Hathirat, N. Kotchabhakdi, L. Missell, and A. Valyasevi. 1989. "Iron Deficiency and Educational Achievement in Thailand." *American Journal of Clinical Nutrition* (suppl.) 50(3): 687–96.

Popkin, B. M., F. S. Solon, T. Fernandez, and M. C. Latham. 1980. "Benefit-Cost Analysis in the Nutrition Area: A Project in the Philippines." *Social Science and Medicine* 14C: 207–16.

SCN News. 1989. *Nutrition in Times of Disaster* 3: 11–13 (UN Administrative Coordinating Committee, Subcommittee on Nutrition, Geneva).

Seshadri, S., and T. Gopaldas. 1989. "Impact of Iron Supplementation on Cognitive Function in Pre-School and School-Aged Children: The Indian Experience." *American Journal of Clinical Nutrition* (suppl.) 50(3): 675–84.

Snodgrass, D. R. 1979. "Economic Aspects." In J. E. Austin, ed., *Global Malnutrition and Cereal Fortification.* Cambridge, Mass.: Ballinger.

Soewondo, S., M. Husaini, and E. Pollitt. 1989. "Effects of Iron Deficiency on Attention and Learning Processes in Preschool Children: Bandung, Indonesia." *American Journal of Clinical Nutrition* (suppl.) 50(3): 667–73.

Sommer, A. 1982. *Nutritional Blindness: Xerophthalmia and Keratomalacia.* Oxford University Press: New York.

Svanberg, U., and A. Sandberg. 1987. "Improved Iron Availability in Weaning Foods Through the Use of Germination and Fermentation." In D. Alnwick, S. Moses, and

U. Schmidt, eds., *Improving Young Child Feeding in Eastern and Southern Africa: Household Level Food Technology*. Proceedings of a workshop in Nairobi, Kenya, October 12–16. Publication IDRC-265E. Ottawa, Canada: International Development Research Centre.

Tilden, R. L., C. R. Pant, G. P. Pokahrel, F. Curtale, R. P. Pokhrel, R. N. Grosse, J. Lepkowski, Muhilal, M. Bannister, J. Gorstein, S. Gorstein-Pak, and Atmarita. 1994. "A Two-year Evaluation Comparing the Impact of Nutrition Education and of Megadose Vitamin A Capsule Distribution on Xerophthalmia, Wasting and Mortality in Nepal." Processed. Duluth, Minn.: The Duluth Clinic.

Toole, M. J. 1992. "Micronutrient Deficiencies in Refugees." *Lancet* 339: 1214–15.

_____, and R. J. Waldman. 1990. "Prevention of Excess Mortality in Refugee and Displaced Populations in Developing Countries." *Journal of American Medical Association* 263(24): 3296–302.

UNHCR (United Nations High Commission on Refugees). 1989. Discussion Paper 1. Technical Support Services. Geneva.

Valyasevi, A. 1988. "Delivery System for Iron Supplementation in Pregnant Women— Thailand Experience." Paper presented at INACG Workshop on Maternal Nutritional Anemia, Washington, D.C., November 14–16. Processed.

Venkatesh Mannar, M. G. 1987. "Control of Iodine Deficiency Disorders by Iodination of Salt: Strategy for Developing Countries." In B. S. Hetzel, J. T. Dunn, and J. B. Stanbury, eds., *The Prevention and Control of Iodine Deficiency Disorders*. New York: Elsevier.

_____. 1993. "Complementarities: Fortification." Paper presented at the United Nations ACC/SCN Micronutrient Forum, WHO, Geneva, February 15–16.

Vital News. 1992. VITAL Project Activities." Vol. 3, no. 1: 7.

Walter, T., I. De Andraca, P. Chadud, and C. Perales. 1989. "Iron Deficiency Anemia: Adverse Effects on Infant Psychomotor Development." *Pediatrics* 84(1): 7–17.

Warren, K. S., D. Bundy, R. Anderson, A. R. Davis, D. A. Henderson, D. T. Jamison, N. Prescott, and A. Senft. 1993. "Helminth Infections." In D. T. Jamison, W. H. Mosley, A. R. Measham, and J. L. Bobadilla, eds., *Disease Control Priorities in Developing Countries*. New York: Oxford University Press for the World Bank.

Weatherall, P. 1988. "The Anemia of Malaria." In W. Werndorfer and I. McGregor, eds., *Malaria Principles and Practices of Malariology*. Edinburgh: Churchill Livingstone.

West, K. P, and A. Sommer. 1987. "Delivery of Oral Doses of Vitamin A to Prevent Vitamin A Deficiency and Nutritional Blindness: A State-of-the-Art Review." ACC/SCN State-of-the-Art Series, Nutrition Policy Discussion Paper 2. United Nations ACC/SCN, Geneva.

WHO (World Health Organization). 1992. "Micronutrient Deficiency Information System—Iodine and Vitamin A." Nutrition Unit, Geneva.

_____. 1988. "Global Status of Vitamin A Deficiency. Vitamin A Deficiency: Time for Action. EPI (Expanded Program on Immunization) *Update*. Geneva, December.

_____. 1992. "National Strategies for Overcoming Micronutrient Malnutrition." Draft Resolution proposed by Rapporteurs of the Executive Board, 89th Session. Geneva.

Yip, R. 1992. Personal communication. Centers for Disease Control, Atlanta, Ga.